Emergency Child and Adolescent Psychiatry

Editor

VERA FEUER

CHILD AND ADOLESCENT PSYCHIATRIC CLINICS OF NORTH AMERICA

www.childpsych.theclinics.com

Consulting Editor
TODD E. PETERS

July 2018 • Volume 27 • Number 3

ELSEVIER

1600 John F. Kennedy Boulevard ● Suite 1800 ● Philadelphia, Pennsylvania, 19103-2899

http://www.theclinics.com

CHILD AND ADOLESCENT PSYCHIATRIC CLINICS OF NORTH AMERICA Volume 27, Number 3
July 2018 ISSN 1056–4993, ISBN-13: 978-0-323-61287-6

Editor: Lauren Boyle
Developmental Editor: Kristen Helm

Child and Adolescent Psychiatric Clinics of North America (ISSN 1056-4993) is published quarterly by Elsevier Inc., 360 Park Avenue South, New York, NY 10010-1710. Months of issue are January, April, July, and October. Business and Editorial Offices: 1600 John F. Kennedy Boulevard, Suite 1800, Philadelphia, PA 19103-2899. Periodicals postage paid at New York, NY and additional mailing offices. Subscription prices are $322.00 per year (US individuals), $594.00 per year (US institutions), $100.00 per year (US students), $382.00 per year (Canadian individuals), $723.00 per year (Canadian institutions), $200.00 per year (Canadian students), $439.00 per year (international individuals), $723.00 per year (international institutions), and $200.00 per year (international students). International air speed delivery is included in all *Clinics* subscription prices. All prices are subject to change without notice. **POSTMASTER:** Send address changes to *Child and Adolescent Psychiatric Clinics of North America*, Elsevier Health Sciences Division, Subscription Customer Service, 3251 Riverport Lane, Maryland Heights, MO 63043. **Customer Service: 1-800-654-2452 (U.S. and Canada); 314-447-8871 (outside U.S. and Canada). Fax: 314-447-8029. E-mail:** JournalsCustomer Service-usa@elsevier.com **(for print support) or** journalsonlinesupport-usa@elsevier.com **(for online support).**

Reprints. For copies of 100 or more of articles in this publication, please contact the Commercial Reprints Department, Elsevier Inc., 360 Park Avenue South, New York, New York 10010-1710 Tel.: 212-633-3874; Fax: 212-633-3820, E-mail: reprints@elsevier.com.

Child and Adolescent Psychiatric Clinics of North America is covered in *MEDLINE/PubMed (Index Medicus), ISI, SSCI, Research Alert, Social Search, Current Contents,* and *EMBASE/Excerpta Medica.*

Contributors

CONSULTING EDITOR

TODD E. PETERS, MD, FAPA
Assistant Chief Medical Informatics Officer/Customer Relationship Manager, Associate
Chief of Staff, Department of Psychiatry and Behavioral Sciences, Vanderbilt University
Medical Center, Medical Director for Inpatient Services, Vanderbilt Psychiatric Hospital,
Assistant Professor of Psychiatry and Behavioral Sciences, Vanderbilt University,
Nashville, Tennessee, USA

EDITOR

VERA FEUER, MD
Director of Emergency Psychiatry and Behavioral Health Urgent Care, Cohen Children's
Medical Center, Donald and Barbara Zucker School of Medicine at Hofstra/Northwell,
New Hyde Park, New York, USA

AUTHORS

ADRIAN JACQUES H. AMBROSE, MD
Clinical Fellow, Department of Psychiatry, Division of Child and Adolescent
Psychiatry, Harvard Medical School, Massachusetts General Hospital, Boston,
Massachusetts, USA

LINDSAY BLITZ, BSN, RN
Clinical Education Specialist, Emergency Department, Connecticut Children's Medical
Center, Hartford, Connecticut, USA

AUSTIN BUTTERFIELD, MD
Senior Instructor, Department of Psychiatry, School of Medicine, University of Colorado,
Medical Director, Psychiatric Emergency Service, Children's Hospital Colorado, Aurora,
Colorado, USA

MARIO CAPPELLI, PhD
Director, Psychiatric and Mental Health Research, Children's Hospital of Eastern Ontario
Research Institute, Associate Professor, Faculty of Graduate and Postdoctoral Studies,
School of Psychology & Department of Psychiatry, University of Ottawa, Ottawa, Ontario,
Canada

DANIELLE CHENARD, BS
Research Associate, Connecticut Children's Medical Center, Hartford, Connecticut, USA

PAULA CLOUTIER, MA
Research Associate, Psychiatric and Mental Health Research, Children's Hospital of
Eastern Ontario Research Institute, Ottawa, Ontario, Canada

DOUGLAS CROOK, BSN, RN
Clinical Coordinator, Behavioral Response Team, Boston Children's Hospital, Boston, Massachusetts, USA

DOREEN DAY, MHSc
Senior Program Manager, The Provincial Council for Maternal and Child Health, Toronto, Ontario, Canada

PATRICIA DICKINSON, RHIT
Health Data Specialist, Center for Care Coordination, Connecticut Children's Medical Center, Hartford, Connecticut, USA

KATHLEEN DONISE, MD
Director, Lifespan Pediatric Behavioral Health Emergency Services, Assistant Professor, Clinician Educator, Department of Psychiatry and Human Behavior, The Warren Alpert Medical School of Brown University, Rhode Island Hospital, Providence, Rhode Island, USA

AMY EGOLF, MD
Chief Fellow, Department of Psychiatry and Human Behavior, The Warren Alpert Medical School of Brown University, Providence, Rhode Island, USA

VERA FEUER, MD
Director of Emergency Psychiatry and Behavioral Health Urgent Care, Cohen Children's Medical Center, Donald and Barbara Zucker School of Medicine at Hofstra/Northwell, New Hyde Park, New York, USA

RUTH GERSON, MD
Assistant Professor, Department of Child and Adolescent Psychiatry, New York University Langone Health, New York, New York, USA

CLARE GRAY, MBA, MD
Associate Professor, Department of Psychiatry, University of Ottawa, Associate Chief, Hospital Based Division Chief, Department of Psychiatry, Children's Hospital of Eastern Ontario, Ottawa, Ontario, Canada

EVA C. HALDANE, PhD
Data Analyst, Child Health and Development Institute of Connecticut, Inc, Farmington, Connecticut, USA

JENNIFER HAVENS, MD
Professor and Vice Chair for Public Psychiatry, Department of Child and Adolescent Psychiatry, New York University Langone Health, Director and Chief of Service, Department of Child and Adolescent Psychiatry, Bellevue Hospital Center, New York, New York, USA

JEFFREY HAWKINS, MSW
Executive Director, Hands TheFamilyHelpNetwork.ca, North Bay, Ontario, Canada

PATRICK J. HEPPELL, PsyD
Clinical Assistant Professor, Department of Child and Adolescent Psychiatry, Hassenfeld Children's Hospital, New York University Langone Health, Child Study Center, Clinical Director of Bellevue Hospital/NYC Administration for Children's Services' Mental Health Team, Nicholas Scoppetta Children's Center, New York, New York, USA

PAMELA HOFFMAN, MD
Assistant Director, Hasbro Psychiatric Emergency Services, Assistant Professor, Clinician Educator, Department of Psychiatry and Human Behavior, The Warren Alpert Medical School of Brown University, Providence, Rhode Island, USA

MONA JABBOUR, MD, MEd
Emergency Medicine Pediatrician, Vice Chief/Chair, Division of Emergency Medicine, Department of Pediatrics, Children's Hospital of Eastern Ontario, Associate Professor, Faculty of Medicine, Department of Pediatrics, University of Ottawa, Ottawa, Ontario, Canada

ALLISON KENNEDY, PhD
Psychologist, Mental Health, Children's Hospital of Eastern Ontario, Ottawa, Ontario, Canada

GARY LELONEK, MD
Child and Adolescent Psychiatrist, Cohen Children's Medical Center, Northwell Health, New Hyde Park, New York, USA

NASUH MALAS, MD, MPH
Assistant Professor, Department of Psychiatry, Division of Child and Adolescent Psychiatry, Assistant Professor, Department of Pediatrics, C.S. Mott Children's Hospital, University of Michigan Hospital System, Ann Arbor, Michigan, USA

ALLISON MATTHEWS-WILSON, LCSW
Clinical Program Specialist, Center for Care Coordination, Connecticut Children's Medical Center, Hartford, Connecticut, USA

JONATHAN MERSON, MD
Medical Director, Behavioral Telehealth, Associate Vice President, Clinical Operations, Behavioral Health Service Line, Assistant Professor, Psychiatry and Emergency Medicine, Donald and Barbara Zucker School of Medicine at Hofstra/Northwell, Glen Oaks, New York, USA

MEGAN M. MROCZKOWSKI, MD
Program Medical Director, Pediatric Psychiatry Emergency Service, Morgan Stanley Children's Hospital, New York Presbyterian Hospital, Assistant Professor of Psychiatry, Columbia University Medical Center, New York, New York, USA

KATE B. O'NEILL, RN, MSN
Director of Clinical Operations, Emergency Medicine Service Line, Northwell Health, New Hyde Park, New York, USA

JEFFREY OESTREICHER, MD
Fellow, Division of Pediatric Emergency Medicine, Cohen Children's Medical Center, Northwell Health, New Hyde Park, New York, USA

CHRISTINE POLIHRONIS, PhD
Research Coordinator, Psychiatric and Mental Health Research, Children's Hospital of Eastern Ontario Research Institute, Ottawa, Ontario, Canada

LAURA M. PRAGER, MD
Director, Child Psychiatry Emergency Service, Transitional Age Youth Clinic, Associate Professor of Child Psychiatry, Division of Child and Adolescent Psychiatry, Harvard Medical School, Massachusetts General Hospital, Boston, Massachusetts, USA

SUCHET RAO, MD
Clinical Assistant Professor, Department of Child and Adolescent Psychiatry, Hassenfeld Children's Hospital, New York University Langone Health, Assistant Director, Psychiatry and Behavioral Health, NYC Administration for Children's Services, New York, New York, USA

JOSHUA A. ROCKER, MD
Associate Chief and Medical Director, Assistant Professor of Pediatrics and Emergency Medicine, Division of Pediatric Emergency Medicine, Cohen Children's Medical Center, Northwell Health, New Hyde Park, New York, USA

STEVEN C. ROGERS, MD, MS-CTR
Attending Physician, Division of Emergency Medicine, Associate Director of Research, Director of Emergency Mental Health Services, Pediatric Emergency Medicine Physician, Connecticut Children's Medical Center, University of Connecticut School of Medicine, Hartford, Connecticut, USA

SUSAN B. ROMAN, RN, MPH
Program Director, Center for Care Coordination, Connecticut Children's Medical Center, Hartford, Connecticut, USA

KRISTINA SOWAR, MD
Assistant Professor, Department of Child and Adolescent Psychiatry, Medical Director of Child Psychiatry Emergency Services, University of New Mexico, Albuquerque, New Mexico, USA

FARA R. STRICKER, FNP-C, RN
Nurse Practitioner, Division of Substance Abuse, Zucker Hillside Hospital, Glen Oaks, New York, USA

DEBORAH THURBER, MD
Child and Adolescent Psychiatrist, Medical Director, Youth and Family Services, Ventura County Behavioral Health, Oxnard, California, USA

KRISTEN TRUFELLI, LMHC
Mental Health Counselor, Behavioral Health Urgent Care Center, Cohen Children's Medical Center, New Hyde Park, New York, USA

MAURA TULLY, MSEd, CCLS
Certified Child Life Specialist, Child Life Department, Cohen Children's Medical Center, New Hyde Park, New York, USA

JOHN W. TYSON Jr, MD
Instructor of Psychiatry, Harvard Medical School, Division of Child and Adolescent Psychiatry, Massachusetts General Hospital, Boston, Massachusetts, USA

JEFFREY J. VANDERPLOEG, PhD
President and CEO, Child Health and Development Institute of Connecticut, Inc, Farmington, Connecticut, USA

Contents

**Preface: Emergency Child and Adolescent Psychiatry: Updates on Evidence Base
and Innovations to Improve Care** xiii

Vera Feuer

The State of Emergency Child and Adolescent Psychiatry: Raising the Bar 357

Megan M. Mroczkowski and Jennifer Havens

The current state of emergency child and adolescent psychiatry includes common historical challenges to safe and effective care as well as recent innovations in multiple settings that increase the quality of that care. These include (1) enhancements within pediatric emergency departments (EDs), (2) specialized and dedicated child psychiatry emergency programs that are hospital based, (3) telepsychiatry programs that spread access to child psychiatric evaluation and treatment planning, and (4) community-based mobile programs diverting youth from EDs. Together, these highlight the work in North America over the past 5 years to improve the care of youth in psychiatric crisis.

**Crisis in the Emergency Department: The Evaluation and Management of Acute
Agitation in Children and Adolescents** 367

Ruth Gerson, Nasuh Malas, and Megan M. Mroczkowski

Acute agitation in children and adolescents in the emergency department carries significant risks to patients and staff and requires skillful management, using both nonpharmacologic and pharmacologic strategies. Effective management of agitation requires understanding and addressing the multifactorial cause of the agitation. Careful observation and multidisciplinary collaboration is important. Medical workup of agitated patients is also critical. Nonpharmacologic deescalation strategies should be first line for preventing and managing agitation and should continue during and after medication administration. Choice of medication should focus on addressing the cause of the agitation and any underlying psychiatric syndromes.

Suicide Evaluation in the Pediatric Emergency Setting 387

Adrian Jacques H. Ambrose and Laura M. Prager

Suicide is 1 of the top 3 leading causes of death in the pediatric population and a serious public health concern. There are evidence-based screening tools for suicide in the pediatric population; however, predicting suicide risks can be a difficult task. The emergency department is an essential source of mental health care for youths and can serve as an important opportunity for suicide screening and subsequent targeted interventions and resource management. More research is needed in emergency department–based screening algorithms and evidence-driven interventions in the pediatric population.

Focused Medical Assessment of Pediatric Behavioral Emergencies   399

Joshua A. Rocker and Jeffrey Oestreicher

> There is no uniformly accepted standard of care for medical clearance of pe-
> diatric patients with psychiatric complaints. Emerging data argue for a thor-
> ough history and physical examination and against routine laboratory
> testing. The differential diagnosis of patients presenting with psychiatric health
> complaints is extensive and includes both medical and psychiatric disorders.
> Providers should remain mindful of anchoring or diagnosis momentum bias
> when caring for these patients, especially patients with a psychiatric history.

An Emergency Department Clinical Pathway for Children and Youth with Mental
Health Conditions   413

Mona Jabbour, Jeffrey Hawkins, Doreen Day, Paula Cloutier,
Christine Polihronis, Mario Cappelli, Allison Kennedy, and Clare Gray

> Children and youth presenting to the emergency department with mental
> health concerns present a challenge for clinicians and system capacity.
> Addressing a significant system gap and sparse strategies in the literature,
> representative leaders from hospital and community agencies developed a
> novel pathway to guide efficient and doable risk assessment and ensure
> timely transition to appropriate community mental health services. This
> article describes and reflects on our innovative Emergency Department
> Clinical Pathway for Children and Youth with Mental Health Conditions
> that bridges traditional barriers between hospital and community settings
> to address mental health needs for this population.

Maintaining Safety and Improving the Care of Pediatric Behavioral Health Patients
in the Emergency Department   427

Fara R. Stricker, Kate B. O'Neill, Jonathan Merson, and Vera Feuer

> Pediatric emergency visits for behavioral health complaints have been
> increasing for more than a decade. There are currently no best practices
> or ideal models of care. However, the evidence base for existing emergency
> department operational concepts can be used to implement modifications
> to workflow, care model, staffing, and physical environment to address pa-
> tient needs. Rapid assessment, split flow, blended care model, multidisci-
> plinary team development, mental health nursing triage, and staff training
> can all positively affect length of stay, staff safety, and patient satisfaction.

Current Pediatric Emergency Department Innovative Programs to Improve the
Care of Psychiatric Patients   441

Susan B. Roman, Allison Matthews-Wilson, Patricia Dickinson,
Danielle Chenard, and Steven C. Rogers

> Emergency departments (EDs) across North America have become a
> safety net for patients seeking mental health (MH) services. The prevalence
> of families seeking treatment of children in MH crisis has become a na-
> tional emergency. To address MH access and improve quality and efficient
> management of children with MH conditions, the authors describe ED pro-
> jects targeting this vulnerable population. Five North American health care
> systems volunteered to feature projects that seek to reduce ED visits and/
> or improve the care of MH patients: Allina Health, Nationwide Children's

Hospital, Children's Hospital of Eastern Ontario, Connecticut Children's Medical Center, and Rhode Island Hospital.

Social Services and Behavioral Emergencies: Trauma-Informed Evaluation, Diagnosis, and Disposition   455

Patrick J. Heppell and Suchet Rao

The emergency department's role in a psychiatric crisis is to assess for safety, provide crisis interventions, reach a diagnosis, make decisions about disposition and treatment, and provide linkage to the next level of care within the hospital or in the community. The evaluation of children and adolescents involved in the child welfare system brings numerous additional challenges to this already complex environment, including familial and systemic issues and an almost ubiquitous history of trauma. This article endeavors to increase the understanding of child welfare–related issues and provides insight toward using a more trauma-informed and comprehensive approach that incorporates all these factors.

Telepsychiatric Evaluation and Consultation in Emergency Care Settings   467

Austin Butterfield

Telepsychiatric care in the emergency setting is a viable and accessible modality that helps address the needs of patients, families, and communities. An expanding literature base for telepsychiatry in multiple clinical settings has shown benefits, including increased access to care, equal efficacy to face-to-face encounters, cost efficiency, decreased wait times, decreased unnecessary psychiatric hospitalizations, and high levels of patient satisfaction. The evidence base for emergency telepsychiatry is growing for pediatric populations. Increased use of the modality is part of the solution to address the high demand for pediatric psychiatric expertise in emergency rooms and to help bridge service gaps in parts of the country.

Psychiatric Community Crisis Services for Youth   479

Kristina Sowar, Deborah Thurber, Jeffrey J. Vanderploeg, and Eva C. Haldane

Each year, increasing numbers of children and families seek care for psychiatric crises; unfortunately, most communities offer limited services to meet these needs. Youth in crisis often present to emergency departments but may not need or benefit from that level of care. Instead, data reflect improved clinical and financial outcomes when communities offer a continuum of crisis services. In this article, the authors present care models from two communities—Ventura County, California, and the state of Connecticut—and review program development, implementation, and monitoring. The authors also highlight principles for leaders to consider in developing these services.

Multidisciplinary Approach to Enhancing Safety and Care for Pediatric Behavioral Health Patients in Acute Medical Settings   491

Gary Lelonek, Douglas Crook, Maura Tully, Kristen Trufelli, Lindsay Blitz, and Steven C. Rogers

Emergency department visits by pediatric behavioral health patients are increasing, increasing the complexity of care. This article describes initiatives at 3 academic medical centers using multidisciplinary teams, including medical, child life, and security staff, to help decrease anxiety and increase patient comfort. Training in Dialectical Behavior Therapy and agitation management simulations increase staff preparedness for working with agitated and emotionally dysregulated patients. Training security personnel and establishing a behavioral health response team ensures that staff members with expertise in managing agitation support the medical teams and patients throughout the hospital.

Training, Education, and Curriculum Development for the Pediatric Psychiatry Emergency Service   **501**

Amy Egolf, Pamela Hoffman, Megan M. Mroczkowski, Laura M. Prager, John W. Tyson Jr, and Kathleen Donise

Pediatric psychiatric emergency care is delivered in different settings with vastly different resources around the country. Training programs lack guidance on developing optimal curricula for this highly variable but crucial setting. A model curriculum for child and adolescent psychiatry trainees may be helpful to provide such guidance; its components include recommendations for assessing baseline knowledge, identifying and teaching core subject content, encouraging development of essential skills, and building in supervision for learners. Future directions include further study in current pediatric emergency psychiatry education and expanding the scope of curricula to include different learners and delivery models.

CHILD AND ADOLESCENT PSYCHIATRIC CLINICS

FORTHCOMING ISSUES

October 2018
Dealing with Death and Dying
David Buxton and Natalie Jacobowski,
Editors

January 2019
**Neuromodulation in Child and
Adolescent Psychiatry**
Jonathan Essary Becker,
Christopher Todd Maley, and
Todd E. Peters, *Editors*

April 2019
**The Science of Well-Being: Integration
into Clinical Child Psychiatry**
Jeffrey Bostic, David Rettew, and
Matthew Biel, *Editors*

RECENT ISSUES

April 2018
Youth Internet Habits and Mental Health
Kristopher Kaliebe and Paul Weigle,
Editors

January 2018
**Co-occurring Medical Illnesses in Child and
Adolescent Psychiatry: Updates and
Treatment Considerations**
Matthew D. Willis, *Editor*

October 2017
Pediatric Integrated Care
Tami D. Benton, Gregory K. Fritz,
and Gary R. Maslow, *Editors*

ISSUE OF RELATED INTEREST

Pediatric Clinics of North America, October 2015 (Vol. 62, No. 5)
Pediatric Prevention
Earnestine Willis, *Editor*
Available at: http://www.pediatric.theclinics.com/

AACAP Members: Please go to www.jaacap.org for information on access to the Child and
Adolescent Psychiatric Clinics. *Resident* Members of AACAP: Special access information is
available at www.childpsych.theclinics.com.

THE CLINICS ARE AVAILABLE ONLINE!
Access your subscription at:
www.theclinics.com

Preface

Emergency Child and Adolescent Psychiatry: Updates on Evidence Base and Innovations to Improve Care

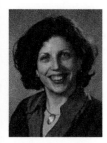

Vera Feuer, MD
Editor

Limited access and fragmentation of mental health care for children and adolescents have been longstanding and well-articulated issues for decades. Increasing suicide rates, especially in the younger age groups, violence in schools, and substance use issues have all been highlighted as particular concerns. Despite receiving much attention of various types, including recommendations by professional organizations, excellent initiatives for screening, as well as collaborative programs with primary care and schools, the number of youths presenting in psychiatric crisis to emergency services continues to increase. Emergency departments also continue to serve as a safety net and as the primary point of entry into the mental health system for many families. There is great variability across the country and across care settings in terms of resources, models of care, and the presence of child psychiatry expertise. The dearth of evidence base, the lack of best practices, and the absence of clinical guidelines impact quality of care and patient outcomes. This issue provides a review of the most salient aspects of the emergency psychiatric care of children and adolescents. We have selected high-yield topics and hope that together they will serve as a helpful guide for anyone working with this population. Each article provides a review of the existing literature and evidence base. Several articles also introduce novel programs where the application of existing evidence and the innovative use of resources have contributed to improving care for this population.

We start by reviewing the current state of affairs in North America and introducing model programs that have successfully "raised the bar" on the standards of care by implementing solutions that provide a framework for the improvement of emergency

Child Adolesc Psychiatric Clin N Am 27 (2018) xiii–xiv
https://doi.org/10.1016/j.chc.2018.04.001
1056-4993/18/© 2018 Published by Elsevier Inc.

childpsych.theclinics.com

services. We continue by reviewing the evaluation and management of the two most common psychiatric emergencies: suicidality and agitation, as well as guidelines for the focused medical assessment of pediatric patients presenting with behavioral emergencies. The subsequent articles on implementing clinical pathways and nursing triage tools in emergency departments include both a literature review and a detailed model program description. We then move on to reviewing the use of multidisciplinary teams to both manage behavioral health patients within acute care settings and transition them to community care. The next articles review solutions for increasing access to care, including emergency telepsychiatry and community crisis programs. There is also a dedicated article on trauma-based approaches, with a special focus on working with foster care youths in crisis. A review of training and education issues and a model curriculum are provided in the final article.

Several remarkable authors from across various institutions were selected for their clinical and research expertise, their innovative programs, and their enthusiasm to share their knowledge. They have been generous in dedicating their time to provide this much-needed review of evidence and guidance regarding these topics. We hope that this issue will fill a gap that exists in the child psychiatry literature and will be helpful in promoting knowledge among child mental health, emergency, and primary care providers alike, as well as offer implementable models and solutions for improving care for our youths in crisis.

Vera Feuer, MD
Division of Emergency Psychiatry
Donald and Barbara Zucker School of Medicine at Hofstra/Northwell
75-59 263rd Street
Glen Oaks, NY 11004, USA

E-mail address:
vfeuer@northwell.edu

The State of Emergency Child and Adolescent Psychiatry: Raising the Bar

Megan M. Mroczkowski, MD[a],*, Jennifer Havens, MD[b,c]

KEYWORDS

- Emergency child and adolescent psychiatry • Systems of care
- Pediatric emergency departments • Telepsychiatry programs
- Child psychiatric evaluation and treatment planning

KEY POINTS

- There are several innovative systems of care in place to care for children and adolescents in psychiatric crisis.
- This article outlines innovations in the pediatric emergency department, specialized child and adolescent psychiatry emergency programs, telepsychiatry programs, and community-based mobile crisis programs.
- These models may serve as inspiration and blueprints for systems-based improvements in child and adolescent psychiatric emergency care throughout North America.

INTRODUCTION

Emergency departments (EDs) struggle with growing numbers of young people presenting in psychiatric crisis that continue to climb, with striking increases in children of younger and younger ages.[1] More specifically, from 2006 to 2011, although all-cause hospitalizations did not increase for children ages 10 to 14, ED visits for mental health conditions increased by 21% and hospitalizations for mental health conditions increased by approximately 50%.[1] Suicide is now the second leading cause of death in adolescents[2] and suicidal ideation and behavior have significantly increased in children and early adolescents presenting to EDs.[1] Coupled with the shrinking capacity for inpatient psychiatric hospitalization, EDs are challenged to safely and effectively manage children in psychiatric crisis, and boarding in EDs and on pediatrics units is

Financial Disclosures: Dr J. Havens serves on the Clinician Advisory Board of Mindyra.
[a] Columbia University Medical Center, 3959 Broadway, MSCH 619C, New York, NY 10032, USA;
[b] Department of Child and Adolescent Psychiatry, NYU Langone Health, One Park Avenue, 7th Floor, New York, NY 10016, USA; [c] Department of Child and Adolescent Psychiatry, Bellevue Hospital Center, 562 First Avenue, 21st Floor, New York, NY 10016, USA
* Corresponding author.
E-mail address: mmm2323@cumc.columbia.edu

Child Adolesc Psychiatric Clin N Am 27 (2018) 357–365
https://doi.org/10.1016/j.chc.2018.02.001
1056-4993/18/© 2018 Elsevier Inc. All rights reserved.

childpsych.theclinics.com

a common occurrence and represents a tremendous burden for children, families, and health care providers.[3–7] Myriad problems underlie the current state of affairs, including reimbursement, work force and parity enforcement limitations, widespread tolerance of substandard care for this population, and the lack of best practices and guidelines.

Historically, the usual model of ED care for young people was evaluation and disposition from a medical emergency room or psychiatric emergency programs serving primarily adults. Although the latter represents a significant advance in adult psychiatric care driven by high volumes of behavioral health patients clogging adult medical EDs, these programs fail to meet the needs of young patients because psychiatric and nursing staff commonly lack child and adolescent expertise and these programs also expose young people to frightening and unsafe environments. Pediatric EDs provide a more child-friendly environment but they lack safe facilities for the management of psychiatric patients, and the medical and nursing staff generally lack sufficient competencies in behavioral health. The challenges of serving young patients in psychiatric crisis in these settings has been well documented.[3,4,6,8] A study in California reports that more than 50% of young people presenting to EDs for self-injurious behavior left without a mental health evaluation.[9]

Fortunately, child and adolescent psychiatrists, health care systems, and state and local governments across North America have begun to mobilize to address the lack of capacity for high-quality psychiatric emergency care for children and adolescents. In 2016, an emergency psychiatry committee was established at the American Academy of Child and Adolescent Psychiatry, which links and supports ED providers across the United States and Canada as they work to improve services in their communities. This is an important development because shared expertise and advocacy are important in moving health care systems to invest resources to develop appropriate services for youth in psychiatric crisis. The delivery of mental health services is associated with low rates of reimbursement relative to medical and surgical services, which presents a barrier to enhancement and expansion in health care systems increasingly motivated by the bottom line. In addition, ED services are generally associated with low collection rates and are justified by the need to fill hospital beds. In an era when contraction or elimination of child psychiatry beds in general hospital settings is the norm, there is little motivation other than quality concerns to invest in these services. Behavioral health disorders, however, are the major morbidity and mortality in an otherwise generally healthy population, children and adolescents. The public health crisis of youth suicidal and self-injurious behavior necessitates pushing health care systems beyond financial calculations and holding them to quality and safety standards that are so central to their mission.[10]

Over the past 5 years, service developments improving the quality of child psychiatric emergency care have been implemented in a variety of arenas, providing a strong framework for dissemination to additional sites. These include adaptations and enhancements to psychiatric emergency care delivered in pediatric EDs, with the development of dedicated space and behavioral health staff as well as the implementation of clinical pathways standardizing assessment, intervention and disposition. This is a basic and first step, acknowledging that the management of behavioral health disorders is part of the central role of pediatric EDs. As volumes and acuity increase, relying on the historically inadequate systems of care must become an aberration rather than the norm. Considerable effort must be made to demand and develop structural reimbursement systems that adequately support emergency psychiatry care in EDs.

In addition, sites with high volumes of ED psychiatric visits (more than 2000 per year) have begun to implement specialized and dedicated programs for the care of youth in psychiatric crisis. These programs require considerable institutional commitment, because they utilize valuable space and require significant financial investment both for buildout and for ongoing operations. Generally, they have required local governmental support and/or philanthropic support for start-up as well as for operations, speaking to the failure of appropriate insurance supports for these crucial services. These programs model the adaptions made to adult psychiatric emergency care, with dedicated and safe spaces and appropriately trained physician, nursing, and social work staff for evaluation, management, and disposition. Extended observation beds, with active treatment, are an important element of these programs, allowing young people who can be stabilized in 3 days to 5 days to avoid longer inpatient admissions. This is critical for children and adolescents, who commonly have their first presentation for behavioral health disorders in EDs.

Third, telepsychiatry is beginning to make important contributions to ED psychiatric care. Given the tremendous shortage of child and adolescent psychiatrists, telepsychiatry presents an opportunity to serve multiple EDs from a centralized site. Large health systems serving multiple hospitals have implemented hub-and-spoke telepsychiatry programs, increasing access to child psychiatric evaluation across care systems, allowing youth to receive appropriate evaluation and disposition planning in EDs without child psychiatry staffing. Compared with treatment as usual, there is evidence from Children's Hospital Colorado that telepsychiatry leads to shorter lengths of stay in EDs (5.5 hours vs 8.3 hours), lower total patient charges ($3493 and $8611), and high patient satisfaction and acceptability.[11] Additionally, a large review demonstrated that telepsychiatry is feasible to implement and that both psychotherapy and psychopharmacology services provided via this modality are possible in the ED setting.[12] Although logistic and reimbursement challenges exist within this model, it is an excellent model for addressing the work force shortage issues.

Finally, mobile programs that provide evaluation and facilitated and effective triage of youth in psychiatric crisis in the community have considerable promise to reduce ED visits. For these programs to be effective, they must have an immediate response capability as well as effective and rapid mental health care in the community.[13] These programs are generally funded by local government investment and provide a viable alternative to EDs for youth at lower levels of acuity and for those families facing challenges in accessing the routine mental health system for their children.

What follows includes examples of these 4 types of program development from across the United States and Canada. Together these programs provide a framework for the development of psychiatric emergency care systems that can be adapted to the needs of specific communities and health care systems. Their implementation represents considerable progress in raising the bar on the standards of care for youth and families in psychiatric crisis.

INNOVATIONS WITHIN PEDIATRIC EMERGENCY DEPARTMENTS: PSYCHIATRIC SERVICES WITHIN PEDIATRIC EMERGENCY DEPARTMENTS, CODE GOLD, FLEXIBLE SPACE IN THE EMERGENCY DEPARTMENT, AND CLINICAL PATHWAYS
Psychiatric Services Within Pediatric Emergency Departments (Nationwide Children's Hospital, Columbus, Ohio)

In response to a sharp increase in behavioral health patient visits to the ED at Nationwide Children's Hospital, the hospital created a new model of care using licensed master's-level behavioral health therapists to complete primary assessments of patients that were then reviewed by phone by a child psychiatry attending physician. Additionally, an ED behavioral health suite was built with 5 safe examination rooms and 1 safe restroom along with a workstation for behavioral health staff. The advantages of this system included providing a safer, quieter place to assess behavioral health patients and dedicated behavioral health staffing.

Nationwide Children's Hospital is also planning on opening the Nationwide Children's Hospital Big Lots Behavioral Health Pavilion in 2020. Although still in the design phase, there are plans for a psychiatric crisis center staffed by an ED physician, psychiatrist, psychiatric and ED nurses, behavioral health clinicians and technicians, and administrative staff. The physical plant blueprints include a medical suite, psychiatric assessment rooms, seclusion room, comfort room, extended observation unit, and crisis phone line.

Code Gold and Flexible Emergency Department Space (Los Angeles County–University of Southern California)

Los Angeles County–University of Southern California (LAC-USC) Hospital has integrated 2 innovative approaches to addressing agitation and lack of space in pediatric EDs. Using the Joint Commission model of codes, LAC-USC uses Code Gold for behavioral health emergencies with a focus on clinical, not security, intervention. When a Code Gold is activated, trained behavioral health nurses and technicians respond en masse to the patient and work to verbally de-escalate the situation. The goal is to address the underlying cause of the agitation and minimize the use of restraints or medications.

Additionally, given the wide fluctuations in volume in pediatric EDs, LAC-USC uses a flexible physical plant model. When the number of behavioral health patients exceeds the safe allotment for a pediatric ED, a portion of the waiting room is temporarily repurposed with stretchers and staffing to support additional patients with behavioral health chief complaints. This model is often used for patients who have been assessed and require inpatient admission and are awaiting an open inpatient bed.

Clinical Pathways for Patients with Autism Spectrum Disorder (Children's Hospital of Philadelphia)

Patients with autism spectrum disorder (ASD) can present to a pediatric ED in a setting of agitation or aggression at home. First and foremost, a medical etiology for this agitation should be considered and ruled out. Common causes for agitation or aggression in adolescents with ASD include constipation, seizures, ear infections, dental infections, pain, sleep problems, undetected injuries, sleep apnea, and urinary tract infections.[14]

At the Children's Hospital of Philadelphia (CHOP), pediatrics created a clinical pathway to optimize the care for patients with ASD who present to the ED with agitation or aggression, many of whom require medical work-up or admission. This clinical pathway is in the public domain, located on the CHOP Web site.[15] Goals of this clinical pathway include facilitating patient compliance and comfort, minimizing patient and staff safety and concerns, and defining a series of practical strategies and methods to organize and structure a patient encounter. The clinical pathway also provides an in-depth description of patients with ASD, including possible clinical features of repetitive behaviors and comorbid conditions.

Communication strategies

- Parents as partners (planning for difficult tasks when parents are present, discussing plan of care in advance of implementing, and frequent 2-way communication with parent and designated staff member)

- Kids care model adaptations (knocking and waiting before entering, allowing for child to become accustomed, introducing self, identifying all at bedside, discussing plan of care, checking name bands, returning in timely manner, and so forth)

- Get low, go slow (getting down to child's level, explaining everything in simple language, breaking down instructions, and positive reinforcement)

- CHOP autism flash cards to help identify people, medical supplies, and procedures using pictures

Environmental modifications

- Sensory sensitivities (tags on clothing, lights, too many people, loud noises, food textures, and too many instructions)

Pain assessment

- Asking patient or parent; often cannot use tools with rating scale or facial expression

- Simplistic language, terms familiar to patient, and minimizing time to focus on pain work best[16]

Given patients with ASD often require a longer ED course to stabilize or may require medical admission and procedures, CHOP has pioneered a new 12-bed medical behavioral unit, co-led by the departments of pediatrics and psychiatry.[17]

Clinical pathways with public health standards of care (Canadian national health care system)

To address increased emergency behavioral health visits and lack of standardized mental health screening tools and pediatric expertise, the Canadian national health care system created an evidenced-based Emergency Department Mental Health Clinical Pathway (EDMHCP) with 2 main goals:

1. Guide risk assessment and decisions on appropriate disposition for children and adolescents who present to an the ED with a behavioral health chief complaint
2. Provide streamlined referral process for follow-up mental health services within community organizations[18,19]

The EDMHCP algorithm begins at triage. Resuscitative/emergent medical care is the initial priority and, once a patient is medically cleared, a mental health screening battery is administered as part of the routine clinical pathway. The patient is subsequently evaluated by a child/youth mental health clinician and ED physician, and the HEADS-ED (Home, Education, Activities and peers, Drugs and alcohol, Suicidality, Emotions and behaviours, and Discharge resources) clinician screening tool is administered. Based on these assessments, the disposition recommendation is determined as in-patient admission, community mental health services, or follow-up with primary care. Community mental health services was further classified as 24-hour rapid response or 7-day response.[18]

Further details of this pathway and its implementation are discussed in Mona Jabbour and colleagues' article, "An Emergency Department (ED) Clinical Pathway for Children and Youth with Mental Health Conditions," in this issue. Both service and process outcomes of EDMHCP are currently being studied with the goals of determining whether or not it improved health care utilization, medical management of behavioral health chief complaints, and coordination of care with outside mental health treatment clinics.[18]

SPECIALIZED CRISIS CENTERS (HOSPITAL BASED): BELLEVUE HOSPITAL CENTER AND UNIVERSITY OF CALIFORNIA, LOS ANGELES

Bellevue Children's Comprehensive Psychiatric Emergency Program

Bellevue Hospital Center in New York has created a system of comprehensive evaluation and management of pediatric psychiatric emergencies, the Children's Comprehensive Psychiatric Emergency Program (CCPEP). After patients are triaged in the pediatric ED, they are transferred to the CCPEP, which includes a 6-bed (4 bedrooms: 2 single rooms and 2 double rooms) extended observation unit providing active treatment, with a nursing station, medical examination room, charting room, waiting room, and 3 offices for evaluation and disposition of patients not meeting criteria for extended observation (danger to self or others or illness impairing safety in the community). This model of care, supported by the New York State Office of Mental Health, allows patients to have a legal status for observation, under Mental Hygiene Law 9.40. This legal status allows child psychiatrists 72 hours in which to evaluate, observe, and re-evaluate patients with the goal of optimal dispositional outcomes.

The CCPEP comprises comprehensive mental health staffing, including child and adolescent psychiatrists, child psychiatry fellows, psychologists, social workers, psychiatry technicians, and psychiatric nurses. The Bellevue CCPEP evaluates more than 2000 patients per year, with 40% meeting criteria for extended evaluation and 60% requiring comprehensive psychiatric and psychosocial evaluation and treatment planning. Dispositional options include discharge home from extended observation with outpatient follow-up (50% of extended observation patients), admission to the Bellevue inpatient child or adolescent psychiatry unit, follow-up in the interim crisis clinic (housed in the CCPEP, allows for close follow-up for patients who do not require admission but would benefit from immediate treatment with facilitated referral to longer-term treatment), and discharge home with referrals to the outpatient clinics (community or hospital based).

Child and Adolescent Psychiatric Emergency Department (University of California, Los Angeles)

In response to 2 sentinel events, Los Angeles County partnered with the City of Los Angeles to create a specialized child and adolescent psychiatric ED. Modeled after the Bellevue CCPEP, Harbor-UCLA is building the first child and adolescent psychiatric ED on the West Coast, scheduled to open in 2018.

This model of care will include dedicated and specialized environment and a firm patient cap after which overflow will go to a pediatric ED. Goals of this new space are to centralize child and adolescent psychiatric emergency care in Los Angeles in 1 location and provide the highest level of patient care with staffing by child and adolescent psychiatrists.

TELEPSYCHIATRY (ZUCKER SCHOOL OF MEDICINE AT HOFSTRA/NORTHWELL HEALTH/LONG ISLAND JEWISH MEDICAL CENTER)

Cohen Children's Medical Center of Northwell Health has a pediatric emergency psychiatry service, which includes a telepsychiatry component. After a 30% increase in ED behavioral health volume from 2011 to 2013, staffing changes were implemented to meet the needs of this vulnerable patient population. Concurrent to the development of an emergency psychiatry service, the Northwell Health system also expanded and included many regional hospitals with varying psychiatric coverage (general psychiatrist, psychiatric nurse practitioner, and no coverage) in the EDs. Telepsychiatry was implemented to provide services to children presenting to other health system hospitals as an alternative to transferring them via emergency medical services or, in some locations, as an alternative to being evaluated by a general psychiatry nurse practitioner/physician provider. As the program expanded to more health system hospitals (they currently there are 14 spoke EDs), the volume of patients requiring telepsychiatric evaluation reached a critical volume and the health system created an independent behavioral telehealth center. The centralized behavioral telehealth center provides comprehensive evaluation and dispositional support with a team of adult and child and adolescent psychiatrists, social workers, case managers, and clerical support associates working together in covering multiple EDs. This telepsychiatry system economizes the highest trained professionals (adult and child and adolescent psychiatrist) in a centralized location, expanding their reach to on-site staff and providing psychiatric care where none is available, allowing for fewer unnecessary transfers and decreased lengths of stay in the EDs.

COMMUNITY MOBILE CRISIS PROGRAMS: EMERGENCY MOBILE PSYCHIATRIC SERVICES (CONNECTICUT CHILDREN'S MEDICAL CENTER)

There are many methods of managing crises within the community, such as triage phone lines, mobile community crisis teams, and local/embedded psychiatric triage teams, all of which are highlighted by Kristina Sowar and colleagues' article, "Psychiatric Community Crisis Services for Youth," in this issue. This article highlights 1 state-wide mobile crisis program from Connecticut. Based on national best practices, this community-based provider network created new goals, clinical benchmarks, and targets for accountability. The goal of the emergency mobile psychiatric services (EMPS) was to respond to psychiatric crises in the community, connect patients to care, and avoid unnecessary ED visits.[13]

The program is funded by Connecticut state grants with third-party reimbursement from Medicaid and commercial insurers.

Any child 18 years of age or younger (19 years of age or younger, if in high school) can access these services. Anyone can call to make a referral to EMPS, by definition the crisis is defined by caller. The only exclusion criteria for EMPS services are for youth currently in psychiatric residential treatment centers, subacute units, or inpatient hospitals.

EMPS undergoes ongoing performance improvement; there are provider performance benchmarks that include high volume, being mobile, and responding within 45 minutes or less. The EMPS team responses to homes, schools, EDs, and communities, and clinical assessment is completed using standardized instruments and follow-up services are put into place within 45 hours. The team has access to psychiatric evaluation and medication management, if needed.

There are more than 16,000 calls annually to the call center, 75% of which are referred on to EMPS. As part of ongoing quality-improvement measures, the EMPS team has calculated that the cost per episode of care is more than $10,000 on the inpatient unit and $842 using EMPS services. EDs can also refer to EMPS, diverting patients from inpatient psychiatric units, and these referrals have saved more than $2 million.[13,20]

SUMMARY

Children and adolescents in crisis or with psychiatric emergencies are growing in number and acuity. This article highlights service developments improving the quality of child psychiatric emergency care that have been implemented in a variety of arenas.

First, innovations within pediatric EDs are described, including clinical pathways for patients with ASD, using Joint Commission Code Gold to optimize clinical staff to de-escalate agitated patients, and clinical pathways with public health standards of care pioneered in Canada. Second, specialized and dedicated units for the evaluation and treatment of children and adolescents in psychiatric crisis at both Bellevue Hospital Center and LAC-USC are outlined. Third, using the Northwell Health/Long Island Jewish Medical Center telepsychiatry program as a model, how telepsychiatry can increase access to child psychiatrists is described. Last, the statewide EMPS in Connecticut is highlighted, a cost-effective and successful means of triaging and treating children and adolescents in crisis in the community, thereby reducing ED visits and inpatient psychiatric hospitalizations.

Together, these 4 areas of care demonstrate myriad innovative and creative means to best care for patients and may be useful to guide system-based improvements for the care of pediatric patients in crisis throughout North America.

ACKNOWLEDGMENTS

The authors would like to thank Drs David Axelson, Paula Cloutier, Vera Feuer, Eron Friedlaender, Charles Glawe, Anik Jhonsa, Patrick Kelly, Erica Shoemaker, and Jeffrey VanderPloeg for sharing information about their respective programs to highlight in this article.

REFERENCES

1. Torio C, Encinosa W, Berdahl T, et al. Annual report on health care for children and youth in the United States: national estimates of cost, utilization and expenditures for children with mental health conditions. Acad Pediatr 2015;15:19–35.
2. Centers for Disease Control and Prevention, National Center for Injury Prevention and Control [Producer]. Web-based Inquiry Statistics Query and Reporting System (WISQARS™): 10 leading causes of death by age group, United States—2013. Available at: http://www.cdc.gov/injury/wisqars/leadingcauses.html. Accessed October 16, 2017.
3. Case S, Case B, Olfson M, et al. Length of stay of pediatric mental health emergency department visits in the United States. J Am Acad Child Adolesc Psychiatry 2011;50:1110–9.
4. Wharff E, Ginnis K, Ross A, et al. Predictors of psychiatric boarding in the pediatric emergency department: implications for emergency care. Pediatr Emerg Care 2011;27:483–9.
5. Mapelli E, Black T, Doan Q. Trends in pediatric emergency department utilization for mental health-related visits. J Pediatr 2015;167:905–10.
6. Sheridan D, Sprio D, Fu R, et al. Mental health utilization in a pediatric emergency department. Pediatr Emerg Care 2015;31:555–9.
7. Grupp-Phelan J, Mahajan P, Foltin GL, et al. The Pediaitrc Emergency Care Applied Research Network: referral and resource use patterns for psychiatric-related visits to pediatric emergency departments. Pediatr Emerg Care 2009;25:217–20.
8. Olfson S, Gameroff M, Marcus S, et al. Emergency treatment of young people following deliberate self-harm. Arch Gen Psychiatry 2005;62:1122–8.
9. Baraff L, Janowicz N, Asarnow J. Survey of California emergency departments about practices for management of suicidal patients and resources available for their care. Ann Emerg Med 2006;48:454–8.
10. Feuer V, Havens J. Teen suicide: fanning the flames of a public health crisis. J Am Acad Child Adolesc Psychiatry 2017;56:723–4.

11. Thomas J, Novins DK, Hosokawa PW, et al. The use of telepsychiatry to provide cost-efficient care during pediatric mental health emergencies. Psychiatr Serv 2018;69(2):161–8.
12. Myers K. American telemedicine association practice guidelines for telemental health with children and adolescents. Telemed J E Health 2017;23(10):779–804.
13. Vanderploeg J, Lu J, Marshall T, et al. Mobile crisis services for children and families: advancing a community-based model in Connecticut. Child Youth Serv Rev 2016;71:103–9.
14. McGonigle J, Venkat A, Beresford C, et al. Management of agitation in individuals with autism spectrum disorders in the emergency department. Child Adolesc Psychiatr Clin N Am 2014;23:83–95.
15. Children's Hospital of Philadelphia. Pathway for the approach to managing behaviors in children with autism spectrum disorder (ASD)/developmental disorders. Available at: http://www.chop.edu/clinical-pathway/autism-spectrum-disorder-developmental-disorders-clinical-pathway. Accessed October 16, 2017.
16. Ely E. Pain assessment of children with autism spectrum disorders. J Dev Behav Pediatr 2016;37(1):53–61.
17. Children's Hospital of Philadelphia. To soothe and heal. 2017. In children's view. Available at: http://www.chop.edu/news/sooth-and-heal. Accessed October 16, 2017.
18. Jabbour M, Reid S, Polihronis C, et al. Improving mental health care transitions for children and youth: a protocol to implement and evaluate an emergency department clinical pathway. Implement Sci 2016;11:1–9.
19. Gerson R. Utilization patterns at a specialized children's comprehensive psychiatric emergency program. Psychiatr Serv 2017;68(11):1104–11.
20. Mroczkowski M, Baroni A, Guanci N, et al. Pediatric psychiatric emergencies: a discussion on systems of care for psychiatric consultation within several hospital systems. Symposium at the American Psychiatric Association 170th Annual Meeting. San Diego, CA, May 20, 2017.

Crisis in the Emergency Department

The Evaluation and Management of Acute Agitation in Children and Adolescents

Ruth Gerson, MD[a],*, Nasuh Malas, MD, MPH[b,c],
Megan M. Mroczkowski, MD[d]

KEYWORDS

• Agitation • Aggression • Restraint/seclusion • Emergency department • Delirium

KEY POINTS

- Acute agitation in children and adolescents in the emergency department carries significant risks to patients and staff and requires skillful management.
- Agitation is a complex symptom, like pain, and effective treatment requires understanding and addressing the multifactorial cause of the agitation, including psychiatric symptoms, physical distress, and environmental triggers.
- Medical work-up of agitated patients is critical to identify and address delirium, catatonia, and pain as sources of agitation. Young children and those with intellectual or developmental disabilities may not be able to verbally report pain or physical distress.
- Nonpharmacologic deescalation strategies should be first line for preventing and managing agitation. These strategies include effective communication, behavioral strategies, risk assessment, multidisciplinary collaboration, and environmental modifications.
- Medications used for treatment of agitation should focus on addressing the cause of the agitation, such as anxiety, delirium, or psychosis, and any underlying psychiatric syndromes, such as autism or attention-deficit/hyperactivity disorder.

Disclosure: Dr R. Gerson receives royalties from American Psychiatric Publishing.
[a] Department of Child and Adolescent Psychiatry, New York University Langone, 462 1st Avenue, New York, NY 10016, USA; [b] Department of Psychiatry, Division of Child and Adolescent Psychiatry, C.S. Mott Children's Hospital, University of Michigan Hospital System, 1500 East Medical Center Drive, L5023, SPC 5277, Ann Arbor, MI 48109-5277, USA; [c] Department of Pediatrics, C.S. Mott Children's Hospital, University of Michigan Hospital System, 1500 East Medical Center Drive, L5023, SPC 5277, Ann Arbor, MI 48109-5277, USA; [d] Department of Psychiatry, Columbia University Medical Center, 3959 Broadway CHONY 6N, New York, NY 10032, USA
* Corresponding author.
E-mail address: Ruth.Gerson@nyumc.org

Child Adolesc Psychiatric Clin N Am 27 (2018) 367–386
https://doi.org/10.1016/j.chc.2018.02.002
1056-4993/18/© 2018 Elsevier Inc. All rights reserved.

childpsych.theclinics.com

INTRODUCTION

Acute agitation in children and adolescents in the emergency department (ED) carries significant risks for patients, families, and staff.[1] The ED environment is rarely designed with agitated patients in mind. The ED presents potentially dangerous objects, a physical layout not conducive to care for agitated patients, a noisy and chaotic milieu, and limited access to therapeutic spaces. The care team may lack the training, resources, or staffing to care for youth with agitation. As a result, opportunities to address agitation early and proactively are missed, often resulting in behavioral escalation, use of physical restraint, patient or staff injury, and disruption to care.

Little has been written on rates of agitation among youth in the ED. Restraint can be used as a proxy for agitation, and one report suggests that 1 in 15 youth presenting to the ED with psychiatric complaints are restrained during the course of their ED stay, with youth with autism experiencing even higher rates of restraint and sedation.[2,3] However, not all youth who are agitated require restraint or sedation, so this proxy likely underestimates the true rate of agitation. As rates of children and adolescents presenting to the ED for psychiatric complaints continue to increase,[4-6] rates of acute agitation and resulting morbidity are likely to increase as well. Children and teens are increasingly presenting to EDs with agitated or aggressive behavior secondary to delirium, psychological trauma, anxiety, intoxication, or underlying behavioral disorders. Other youth being seen for other psychiatric or physical health concerns may become agitated because of pain, physical discomfort, or poor distress tolerance, exacerbated by overstimulation, long wait times, or lack of privacy.

Providers struggle with management of agitation in the ED. At times, treatment decisions may be reactive and predicated more on provider comfort than an etiologically focused approach to pediatric agitation management.[7] ED providers may turn to anesthetic drugs such as ketamine, midazolam, and barbiturates for rapid sedation of agitated youth, despite the potential for neurotoxicity and neurodevelopmental sequelae.[8,9] In addition, patients with agitation can disrupt the milieu in the ED, affecting the care of youth and families in adjoining rooms or in the general ED environment, particularly when the acuity of the ED is high. Child psychiatrists should educate, support, and guide ED staff in effective and safe management of agitation, using both nonpharmacologic and pharmacologic strategies.

Understanding Agitation in Children and Adolescents in the Emergency Department

Agitation, like pain and so many other acute symptoms, is multifactorial. It is much like a vital sign, signaling distress and dysfunction in the patient warranting evaluation and management. It can range from overblown tantrums to psychotic dysregulation. Often agitation is reactive, occurring in response to a perceived provocation or stressor. Rarely, agitation and aggression may be premeditated and purposeful. Agitation stems from a complex interplay of individual, physical, and environmental risk factors[10-12] (**Box 1**). Even a child without obvious risk factors can become agitated in the setting of fear, discomfort, pain, and the stressful environment of the ED. All patients who enter the ED should be evaluated for risk of agitation both initially and in an ongoing way. The ED team should work proactively to mitigate any modifiable risk factors, reduce environmental triggers, and provide deescalation when needed. The management of agitation should be individualized to the specific needs of each patient and the causal factors behind the agitation.

Clinicians faced with a patient manifesting acute agitation may have limited time for evaluation, but even a momentary appraisal of the patient and the chart can provide

---

Box 1
Risk factors for development of agitation and aggression in youth

Nonmodifiable risk factors:

- Past history of aggression (particularly violence within 24 hours before presentation)
- History of property destruction
- History of physical or sexual abuse
- History of interpersonal violence
- History of previous psychiatric hospitalization
- History of previous disciplinary action at school/other environments
- Traumatic brain injury
- Developmental delay/cognitive delay
- Male gender
- Low family income
- Criminal history or gang involvement

Modifiable risk factors:

Psychological factors
- Impulsivity
- Poor distress tolerance
- Limited insight
- Difficulty establishing trust in others
- Negative world view
- Lack of empathy
- Difficulty with authority figures

Psychiatric factors:
- Disruptive behavior disorder
- Conduct disorder
- Autism spectrum disorder
- Severe anxiety, irritability or mood lability
- Psychotic disorder
- Delirium
- Catatonia
- Substance use, intoxication or withdrawal (particularly at early age)

Physical health factors:
- Central nervous system disorders
- Metabolic disorders
- Endocrine disorders
- Genetic disorders
- Acute or chronic pain
- Poor sleep
- Inflammation or infection

Data from Refs.[10,13–24]

---

key information that is necessary for management, and can be feasible in any circumstance. The briefest assessment should still include focused review of presenting history, past diagnoses and past episodes of agitation (including triggers and response to intervention), and vitals. Assessment starts from the first moments of observation. Even if the child is agitated on arrival, clinicians can assess the developmental level, use of language, and physical appearance, while obtaining a clinical history, developmental history, and identification of triggers or contextual factors from accompanying adults. The goal is to glean information as quickly and efficiently as possible to best understand the potential antecedent factors precipitating and perpetuating the patient's presentation of agitation.

Determining the cause of agitation continues with an assessment of the child's response to intervention. Evaluation must also be ongoing, because triggers for agitation can evolve over time. Quickly understanding the cause of, and triggers for, agitation requires a multidisciplinary approach. The bedside nurse is uniquely suited to notice changes in the patient's mental status or behavior, engage crisis services when needed, and implement nonpharmacologic interventions early. Family members can provide a premorbid developmental and behavioral baseline of their child and identify recent cognitive, emotional, and behavioral changes. Collateral information from other key sources, such as outpatient providers or school staff, is helpful when possible.

The physical examination can be critical in identifying factors contributing to agitation.[10] Regardless of the acuity of the situation, the physical examination should not be overlooked because it aids in guiding intervention and preventing recurrence of agitation. If the child is uncooperative with examination, visual assessment of gait, pupil size, general appearance, and review of recent vital signs can provide important clues to physical or genetic disease, intoxication, and developmental/functional disability. A focused head-to-toe evaluation should assess for possible head trauma, hemotympanum, neck stiffness, vision and hearing deficits, dental ailments, signs of infection or cardiorespiratory decompensation, evidence of peripheral or central nervous system dysfunction, and any localized pain. Laboratory and imaging evaluation should be guided by clinical history, physical examination, symptom evolution, and thoughtful clinical judgment.

Nonpharmacologic Approaches to Prevention and Management of Agitation

In parallel to the evaluation process, nonpharmacologic strategies for preventing and deescalating agitation should be used. Environmental, communication, and behavioral interventions are the first line of agitation management.[25–27] Use of medications does not preclude use of these nonpharmacologic interventions and they can be used simultaneously. Often, the use of nonpharmacologic interventions can obviate medication. If medications are still required, the use of nonpharmacologic interventions can allow decreased dosing or frequency of pharmacotherapy, or mitigate the potential psychological trauma that can be experienced with involuntary medications or restraint.

Early recognition

Early recognition of agitation risk is key to prevention. Clinicians rarely screen for or systematically predict agitation, especially in youth presenting with nonviolent psychiatric or physical complaints.[28,29] Few studies have shown screening or assessment tools to proactively anticipate risk of agitation in the ED setting, especially in youth[13,30–33] (**Table 1**).

In the absence of concrete screening tools, risk assessment should include talking to the patient and family about warning signs and triggers for behavioral escalation, as well as calming strategies. For example, rocking in a young child may represent a self-soothing strategy that should be supported to allow for deescalation, but in another child may represent an early warning sign for eventual aggressive behavior. Assessing developmental level aids identification of developmentally appropriate warning signs and soothing tools. Advance communication and preparation with families allows ED clinicians to recognize and stem the progression of agitation.[61]

Environmental strategies to prevent and deescalate agitation

The ED environment is busy, stimulating, and unpredictable. High levels of ambient noise and smells, variability in lighting and temperature, physical stimuli (pain, fatigue,

Table 1
Screening and assessment tools for pediatric agitation and aggression

Scales	Items	Domains Assessed	Scoring	Interpretation
Dynamic Appraisal of Situational Aggression (DASA)	7	• Irritability • Impulsivity • Unwillingness to follow instructions • Sensitive to perceived provocation • Easily angered • Negative attitudes • Verbal threats	• Scored 0 (absent) or 1 (present) • Measures over past 24 h	• Each increase in score, increases likelihood of agitation by factor of 1.77 • Some use cutoff score of 4 • Lower predictive validity in youth
Brief rating of Aggression by Children and Adolescents (BRACHA 0.9)	14	• Personal history of aggression • Personal risk factors for aggression • Past violence, impulsivity in the emergency room	• Responses are yes/no to presence or absence of qualities • Measures over past week	• Items weighted • Age factored into score • Cutoff for risk of any aggression is 13 • Maximums score of 32 • All items predictive (P<.007) • Good predictive value (ROC of 0.75 for aggression) and inter-rater reliability
Modified Overt Aggression Scale (OAS)[a]	4	• Verbal aggression • Aggression toward property • Aggression toward self • Physical aggression toward others	• Severity and frequency rated from 0–4 with prompts provided • Measures over past week	• Items weighted with greater weight toward physical aggression • Maximum score of 40
Children's Aggression Scale (CAS) Parent and Teacher Forms	33	• Verbal aggression • Aggression toward objects/animals • Provoked physical aggression • Unprovoked physical aggression • Use of weapons	• 5-point scale with increasing frequency and severity from "never" to "most days" • Multiple informants • Measures over past year	• Items weighted on severity with cutoffs • Provided T scores and percentiles • Excellent internal consistency (0.93)
Aggression Questionnaire (AQ)	34	• Physical aggression • Hostility • Verbal aggression • Indirect aggression • Anger	• No specified time period for assessment • 5-point scale from "not at all like me" to "completely like me"	• Total score along with inconsistent responding index • Cutoffs for severity • Excellent internal consistency (0.89) • Test-retest reliability of 0.80

Abbreviation: ROC, receiver operating characteristic.
[a] Scales are free to the public.
Data from Refs.[13,34–60]

hunger), boredom, and frequent interaction (including touch and invasive interventions) with strangers can all trigger agitation.[10,62,63] Children with intellectual disability (ID), autism spectrum disorder, impulsivity, attention deficits, or low frustration tolerance can be particularly susceptible to distress from these environmental stimuli.[62,64–67]

The initial ED assessment of every patient should include ascertaining any particular sensitivities or sensory triggers. It can be helpful to have a member of the care team meet with family early in the ED process to develop a crisis management plan and identify ways to make the environment as therapeutic as possible. Simple interventions such as turning down lights, canceling unnecessary interventions (eg, frequent vital signs checks or intravenous (IV) hep-locks), moving the child to an area where it is possible to move freely unperturbed, or offering preferred sensory tools or distraction techniques (such as an iPad or a favorite cartoon) may prevent escalation. Creating consistency across the care team is also important to prevent agitation, particularly for children with anxiety disorders, developmental delays, or autism.[61,62] Small interventions like the use of a visible schedule can reduce anxiety. Providers should identify themselves and their role on the care team and warn the child in advance about any touch or physical interventions. Demonstrating the examination on an accompanying adult can be helpful. Communication about plans, expectations, and rules should be consistent across all providers.

If the child does escalate, the child should be moved to a calming, safe environment within the ED, away from other patients.[22] Access to any potentially dangerous objects should be restricted.[22] Many EDs now include specialized areas for psychiatric treatment, or dual-purpose rooms where medical equipment mounted on the wall can quickly be secured and locked. Although additional staff should be called for support and safety, 1 staff member or provider should be identified as the key contact for the child, and another as liaison to the family.

Communication strategies for deescalating agitation
Effective communication is important for all aspects of agitation management. Many youth have specialized communication needs that may not be immediately recognized by ED staff. Visual or adaptive communication tools such as visual cue boards, mobile devices, sign language, or interpreter services for children with limited English proficiency can help patients and staff identify needs and address problems.[61]

Communication with the child should be provided in a neutral, empathic tone. Often, getting down to the patient's eye level, speaking in a soft and inviting tone with clear, concrete, and simple language makes it easier for the child to process information or follow through with requests. Body language should be respectful, nonconfrontational, and relaxed but confident and without sudden movement or intrusions into personal space.[22] Simply asking "How can I help?" in a sincere tone can often deescalate an agitated child. Children often struggle to articulate their needs and emotions when upset, so reflecting emotions, asking closed-ended questions, or making thoughtful hypotheses ("You seem really upset, and I wonder if it's related to…") can help children identify their needs. Offer choices (eg, of snack or television channel) to allow the child to feel some semblance of control, while setting clear and nonjudgmental limits. Repetition may be needed to give agitated children time to process and to assure them that they are being heard.

Family engagement
Family plays a critical role in the prevention and nonpharmacologic management of agitation. Caregiver involvement has been shown to reduce anxiety and behavioral

escalation in all patients, particularly those with cognitive delays or autism.[21,61] Families can provide reassurance and comforting physical touch, or provide comforting items from home to sooth the child while in the ED. In some circumstances, family members or other visitors may antagonize the child, or be a primary factor in the cause of the child's agitation.[22] In those cases, brief respite from the family member or visitor may be therapeutic for the patient. The care team can also model effective communication and behavioral techniques for the family, thus educating families on ways to parent disruptive patient behaviors in the future. In particular, praise for adaptive behaviors, as well as validation of the patient's emotions, can be highly effective in preventing behavioral escalation but also in the deescalation of agitation. Witnessing this modeled effectively can be a powerful tool for a family, especially when so much focus is placed on the negative behaviors and qualities of a child's presentation.

Behavioral strategies for deescalation of agitation
Distraction techniques, child life services, social engagement, and cognitive behavior therapy can mitigate anxiety and enhance the child's ability to cope with distress in the ED environment.[68,69] Coping kits can also be developed in advance for children with specific needs, such as children with autism, severe anxiety, or developmental delay.[61] These kits may include sensory tools (a soft textured ball or fidget spinner), premade schedules, and short stories to help the child acclimate to the ED. Small prizes or a token economy can incentivize positive behavior and enhance motivation for the child to engage in care, especially for younger children.

Restraint and seclusion
Use of restraint and seclusion should be reserved only for when nonpharmacologic strategies, management of physical health comorbidities, and cause-focused medication use are unsuccessful in curbing agitation and the patient poses an imminent threat of harm to self or others.[21,22,25] Restraint and seclusion can result in significant psychological trauma or even physical injury to the patient and should be used only as a last resort to ensure patient safety.[25,70–72] Furthermore, the process of restraint and seclusion can be a high-risk period for staff or provider injury and therefore proactive interventions to mitigate the need to pursue restraint and seclusion can aid in reducing the risk of staff harm.[72] Close monitoring should be used with the use of quality indicators to ensure that the use of restraint and seclusion is heavily monitored and mitigated when possible.[21,25]

Psychopharmacologic management of agitation
There are well-established, evidence-based consensus guidelines for psychopharmacologic management of agitation or aggression in adult patients in the ED, namely the Consensus Statement of the American Association for Emergency Psychiatry Project BETA (Best Practices in Evaluation and Treatment of Agitation) Psychopharmacology Workgroup.[73] Project BETA asserts that a combination of verbal deescalation, medication, and environmental modifications can decrease the need for restraint in the ED.[74] Project BETA also emphasizes that the choice of medication for agitation should be individualized and based on an assessment of the cause of agitation. These principles are true for youth as well, but the pathophysiology of agitation and vulnerability to adverse drug effects in youth are often different compared with adults.

The differential diagnosis for pediatric agitation in the ED is broad. Potential environmental triggers should be addressed first, through the strategies identified earlier. Once environmental triggers have been addressed, it can be helpful to consider a few broad categories of potential causal factors: physical disease; delirium (including substance intoxication or withdrawal); autism and developmental disabilities; psychosis and mania; and other psychiatric disorders, including agitated catatonia, disruptive behavior disorders, anxiety, and depression. If the cause of agitation is unknown, the early assumption should be that the cause is related to a general medication condition or intoxication, or multifactorial, unless shown to be otherwise.[10,25]

Medication for agitation should be used when initial nonpharmacologic methods of deescalation have been unsuccessful in calming a patient, and intervention is necessary for safety. The goals of pharmacotherapy for agitation include (1) treating the underlying cause of distress, and (2) calming the patient sufficiently to effectively and accurately provide assessment and treatment,[21] which includes providing medication that is fast acting, calming, but not overly sedating, while mitigating the risk of adverse drug effects.[21] Oral medication should be offered preferentially to intramuscular (IM) or IV medication. If a patient is already in psychiatric treatment, carries a well-established diagnosis, and is on historically beneficial medication, this can guide the choice of medication used in a crisis. For example, a child with attention-deficit/hyperactivity disorder (ADHD) who is on clonidine for impulsivity and agitation may benefit from an additional smaller or equivalent dose of clonidine when agitated. When considering new medications, ED providers must also be careful to avoid drug interactions and adverse drug effects.

Types of Medication Used for Agitation

Antihistamines, benzodiazepines, and neuroleptics are the medications most often used to treat acute agitation in children and adolescents in the ED. At some centers, alpha-2 agonists are also used for some forms of agitation and behavioral escalation. General recommendations regarding each medication class and evidence regarding their use for acute agitation management in the ED pediatric population are highlighted later (**Table 2**).

Diphenhydramine

Diphenhydramine is widely used for agitation in ED settings, but there has been only 1 randomized controlled trial of diphenhydramine versus placebo for agitation in children. This study showed no significant difference between the two medications, with the IM route being more effective than the oral route.[75] No studies have assessed the effectiveness of diphenhydramine in ED settings. Retrospective review of as-needed (PRN) medication efficacy on an inpatient unit found that diphenhydramine was effective in 36% of cases, compared with efficacy of neuroleptics in 33% of cases and benzodiazepines in 12% of cases, although this study was not placebo controlled.[76] Patients administered diphenhydramine should be monitored for paradoxic reactions, including worsening agitation and disinhibition, as well as for delirium, especially if receiving other anticholinergic medications.

Benzodiazepines

Benzodiazepines are also widely used for agitation in the ED given their anxiolytic effect. Despite their widespread use, there have been no randomized controlled trials of benzodiazepines for this specific indication. Use of benzodiazepines should be avoided in young children and some youth with autism/because of the risk for paradoxic reactions.

Neuroleptics

Several studies on PRN neuroleptic use relate to the use of IM ziprasidone compared with other neuroleptics. A retrospective chart review compared IM ziprasidone with IM

Table 2
Medications and dosing guidance for pediatric agitation and aggression

	Medication	Dosing	Onset of Action	Peak Effect	t₁/₂	Potential Side Effects
Antihistamine	Diphenhydramine (PO, LIQ, IM, IV)	12.5–50 mg Or 1 mg/kg/dose	Oral: 1 h	Oral: 2 h	5 h 24 min	Paradoxic worsening Sedation Avoid in delirium
	Hydroxyzine (PO)	12.5–50 mg	1 h	2 h	7 h 6 min	Paradoxic worsening Orthostasis Sedation Avoid in delirium
Alpha-2 Agonists	Clonidine (PO)	0.05–0.1 mg	30 min–1 h	2–4 h	12–16 h	Hypotension/bradycardia Orthostasis Rebound hypertension/ tachycardia Sedation
Benzodiazepine	Lorazepam (PO, IM, IV)	0.5–2 mg Or 0.05–0.1 mg/kg/dose	Oral: 1 h IV: 1–5 min IM: 20–30 min	Oral: 2 h IM/IV: <25 min	10–20 h	Paradoxic worsening Sedation Respiratory suppression Do not coadminister IV/IM lorazepam with IM olanzapine because of risk of respiratory suppression

(continued on next page)

Table 2
(continued)

Neuroleptic	Medication	Dosing	Onset of Action	Peak Effect	$t_{1/2}$	Potential Side Effects
	Haloperidol (PO, IM, IV)	0.5–5 mg (IM half dose of oral) Or 0.55 mg/kg/dose	Oral: 1 h IM/IV: <5 min	Oral: 2–6 h IM/IV: 20 min	Oral: 15–30 h IM: 20 h IV: 14–26 h	EPS QT prolongation (IM, IV) Hypotension
	Chlorpromazine (PO, IM)	12.5–50 mg (IM half dose of oral) Or 0.55 mg/kg/dose	Oral: 30–60 min IM: 15 min	Oral: 30–60 min IM: 15 min	7–8 h	QT prolongation Hypotension Sedation
	Olanzapine (PO, SL, IM)	Oral: 2.5–10 mg IM should be 1/4 PO dose	Oral: 5 h IM: 15–45 min	Oral: 5 h IM: 15–45 min	21–51 h	Metabolic risk Orthostasis Sedation Do not coadminister IV/IM lorazepam with IM olanzapine because of risk of respiratory suppression
	Ziprasidone (PO, IM)	10–20 mg oral 5–10 mg IM	Oral: 6 h IM: 15 min	Oral: 7 h IM: 1 h	3–4 h	Oral should be given with fatty foods EPS QT prolongation Orthostasis Sedation
	Risperidone (PO, SL)	0.25–1 mg Or 0.005–0.01 mg/kg/dose	<1 h	1 h	3–20 h	EPS Metabolic risk Sedation Orthostasis
	Quetiapine (PO)	25–50 mg Or 1–1.5 mg/kg/dose divided	<1 h	30 min–2 h	5 h	Sedation Hypotension

Abbreviations: EPS, extrapyramidal symptoms; LIQ, liquid; PO, oral; SL, sublingual; $t_{1/2}$, half-life; TD, transdermal.

olanzapine and showed that aggression decreased in 90.2% of patients receiving olanzapine and 84.9% of patients receiving ziprasidone. Ziprasidone patients received significantly more emergency medications.[77] A second case-controlled, retrospective chart review compared the combination of IM haloperidol with IM lorazepam and IM ziprasidone.[78,79] This study found no significant difference between these two regimens in terms of restraint duration, use of rescue medications, or vital sign changes.[78] Although these studies are compelling, a survey of expert child and adolescent psychiatrists working in consult-liaison and ED settings indicated that none would identify ziprasidone as first line for agitation in the ED because of concerns for cardiac effects and effects on metabolism depending on nutritional status (Gerson, 2018, unpublished data).

Despite their widespread use for this indication, 1 systematic review and meta-analysis of second-generation neuroleptics for treatment of disruptive or aggressive behavior in youth with average intelligence showed only risperidone had moderate-quality to high-quality evidence supporting its use for this indication. There was low-quality evidence to support other neuroleptics or mood stabilizers.[80] However, risperidone, olanzapine, haloperidol, and chlorpromazine are frequently used as PRN medications for agitation in the ED, especially for youth with severe agitation/aggression, mania or psychosis, alcohol intoxication, and delirium. Caution should be taken with the risk for extrapyramidal symptoms (EPS), especially acute dystonic reactions and akathisia, as well as monitoring of corrected QT, blood pressure, heart rate, and orthostasis. Particular caution should be taken with the use of olanzapine because there is risk for cardiorespiratory suppression with coadministration of olanzapine with benzodiazepines, especially with parenteral administration.

Choosing Medication for a Patient with Agitation

Pharmacologic treatment should target the underlying causal factor when possible. Use of medication should be integrated into a broader treatment plan of behavioral and environmental strategies and verbal deescalation. Common diagnoses associated with acute agitation with corresponding psychopharmacology considerations are outlined later (**Table 3**).

Attention-deficit/hyperactivity disorder

Youth with ADHD may be more likely to become agitated in the ED in the evenings as stimulant medications wear off, or if regular doses of medications are missed while waiting in the ED. Querying whether a child with ADHD has missed home medication and administering it in the ED (avoiding late-afternoon or evening dosing of stimulants), or considering a dose of an alpha-2 agonist, can provide cause-focused treatment. Nonpharmacologic interventions (such as distraction techniques and engagement in soothing, meaningful activities) can be very helpful as well. Diphenhydramine may be effective in younger children. Neuroleptics may be warranted if the child is actively aggressive or if other nonpharmacologic and pharmacologic strategies are ineffective, although it should be remembered that the EPS risk is higher in youth not experiencing a manic or psychotic episode.

Psychosis

In adolescents or young adults with psychotic disorders, neuroleptics are often first-line treatment, including for acute agitation in the context of psychosis. It is imperative that the diagnostic assessment be reviewed and clarified to ensure that the child truly has a psychotic disorder because other confounding diagnoses may include severe

Table 3
Evaluation and management considerations based on potential cause affecting pediatric agitation

Cause	Considerations	Nonpharmacologic Approaches	Pharmacologic Considerations[a]
ADHD	• Reduced effect of stimulant in late afternoon and evening • Environmental triggers	• Distraction techniques • Engage in meaningful activities • Use of calming strategies that have historically been helpful	• Stimulant • Alpha-2 agonists • Diphenhydramine[b] • Neuroleptics (if aggressive)
Psychosis	• Clarify diagnosis and contributing causal factors • Assess for catatonia • Assess for comorbid anxiety or psychological trauma • Assess and monitor physical health	• Minimize overstimulation • Provide a structure and routine • Clarify roles of care team members and care being provided • Provide a quiet, calm, private environment • Monitor for any comorbid pain or discomfort and treat	• Neuroleptics • Lorazepam
Autism spectrum disorder and intellectual disability	• Assess ability to communicate needs and emotions • Assess developmental needs • Assess and monitor physical health	• Minimize overstimulation • Attempt to enhance communication via visuals, use of caregivers and using communication strategies that historically work • Provide structure and routine • Use calming strategies that are historically helpful • Be aware of sensory needs	• Benzodiazepines[b] • Diphenhydramine[b] • Alpha-2 agonists • Neuroleptics
Delirium	• Conduct a thorough evaluation of clinical and pharmacologic factors influencing presentation (**Table 4**) • Minimize use of benzodiazepines, opioids and anticholinergics • Be aware of developmental and psychiatric baseline	• Provide regular verbal reassurance • Continually reorient the patient • Provide familiar objects, comfort from home • Engage caregivers in deescalation strategies • Minimize overstimulation • Address any sensory deprivation • Provide a quiet, calm, private environment • Ensure patient is in appropriate care setting and strongly consider transfer to medical ED setting	• Neuroleptics • Alpha-2 agonists

(continued on next page)

Table 3
(continued)

Cause	Considerations	Nonpharmacologic Approaches	Pharmacologic Considerations[a]
Catatonia	• Assess for both medical and psychiatric contributors to presentation, particularly past history of autism, developmental delay, mood disorders, or neurologic disease	• Minimize overstimulation • Provide a quiet, calm, private environment • Engage caregivers in deescalation strategies • Ensure patient is in appropriate care setting and strongly consider transfer to medical ED setting	• Lorazepam (often at high dose and frequency)
Substance intoxication or withdrawal	• Assess physical health closely, including medical comorbidities and medical stability • Obtain toxicologic work-up, including consideration of gas chromatography mass spectrometry	• Minimize overstimulation • Provide verbal reassurance, reorientation if evidence of comorbid delirium • Use calming strategies that are historically helpful • Ensure patient is in appropriate care setting and strongly consider transfer to medical ED setting	• Benzodiazepines • Neuroleptics (if aggressive) • Alpha-2 agonists

Be aware that the patient may be nonadherent to medication regimen or may have missed doses while waiting in the ED. Restarting the patient's home medication regimen or ensuring patients are receiving their home regimens can be helpful.

[a] Consider providing the patient with an extra dose or half dose of their home psychotropic if currently on a beneficial home psychotropic regimen.

[b] Be aware that these psychotropic agents have a potential for paradoxic reactions (worsening of anxiety, neuroexcitation, worsening agitation), particularly with this population.

anxiety/obsessive-compulsive disorder, intrusive thoughts in children with autism or ID, psychological trauma or posttraumatic stress disorder, delirium, and traumatic brain injury.

If the patient is already on a neuroleptic, an extra dose of the same agent may be considered to avoid polypharmacy, although this is not always feasible because of drug formulation, onset of action, or risk of toxicity. Lorazepam may be added for additional anxiolytic effect for highly agitated patients while being cautious about respiratory suppression (especially with olanzapine) or hypotension. Also, diphenhydramine or benztropine can be added if the patient has a history of or emergent extrapyramidal side effects. Although pharmacologic interventions are being pursued, remember that perceptual disturbances may be worsened by the chaos and overstimulation of the ED. Moving the patient to a quiet and private area can be powerfully calming. Other youth may not be able to express physical discomfort (including iatrogenic effects such as dystonia) because of disorganized thinking and speech. Physical assessment and treatment should not be neglected.

Table 4
Critical care acronym: causes for evaluation and monitoring of pediatric delirium

Cardiovascular	Anemia, shock, vasculitis, hypertensive encephalopathy
Respiratory	Respiratory insufficiency, respiratory failure, pneumothorax
Infection	Sepsis, encephalitis, urinary tract infection, meningitis, fever, pneumonia, tracheitis, cellulitis/skin breakdown, surgical site infection
Toxins	Polypharmacy, heavy metals, drug-drug interactions
Inflammatory process	Autoimmune and rheumatologic disease
CNS disorder	Stroke, seizure, head trauma, intracranial bleed, tumor, anoxic injury
Abuse/withdrawal	Alcohol, benzodiazepines, opioids, barbiturates
Liver	Liver insufficiency, liver failure, hyperammonemia
Constipation	
Alimentation	Electrolyte imbalance, nutritional deficiencies, dehydration
Renal	Renal insufficiency or failure
Endocrinopathies	Glycemic disturbance, thyroid disease, parathyroid disease, adrenal disease

Abbreviation: CNS, central nervous system.

From Malas N, Brahmbhatt K, McDermott C, et al. Pediatric delirium: evaluation, management and special considerations. Curr Psychiatry Rep 2017;19(9):65; with permission.

Autism spectrum disorder and intellectual disability

Youth with autism and ID have a greater rate of physical and psychiatric symptoms and use the ED more frequently than their peers without autism or ID.[64] Youth with autism and/or ID may also be less able to communicate pain, anxiety, discomfort, hunger, or physical needs, which may lead to or be confused with agitation. If medication is required, benzodiazepines and antihistamines should be used cautiously given the risk of paradoxic reaction. Parents should also be asked about the response to these agents in the past. Clonidine, risperidone, or chlorpromazine can also be used. IM administration should be avoided whenever possible. Although aripiprazole is US Food and Drug Administration approved for irritability and aggression in youth with autism, this is less commonly used for acute agitation given the risk for activation and akathisia.

Delirium

Delirium is the clinical manifestation of disturbances in the homeostatic milieu of the brain resulting in acute global central nervous system dysfunction.[81,82,83,84] All patients with agitation should be screened for delirium either through clinical assessment or through formal screening. Medical work-up for delirium is beyond the scope of this article (see **Table 4**). The first step in addressing delirium is a thorough systems-based reviewed of underlying medical causes contributing to delirium and treating these causes. Reduction or discontinuation of potential offending agents should be, when possible, the initial approach of pharmacologic management. Benzodiazepines, anticholinergics, and opioid analgesics should be avoided, weaned, or limited. Medications may be needed to address underlying causes potentiating delirium, such as pain or active clinical disease, while also being considered for use in managing the sequelae of delirium, such as sleep-wake disturbance and agitation.

Neuroleptics are the most commonly used pharmacologic intervention for symptomatic management of delirium.[85] Choice of neuroleptic agent should account for the particular needs of a given patient, including route of administration, time to effect, potential side effects, illness factors, and the specific symptoms of delirium being targeted. Haloperidol has largely been replaced by second-generation neuroleptics as the first-line agents with fewer side effects and comparable efficacy.[86,87] Risperidone, olanzapine, and quetiapine are the most commonly used neuroleptics for delirium management in youth.[86,88]

Catatonia

Catatonia can occur in the context of both medical and psychiatric illness, and is not confined to psychotic illnesses. It is much more commonly seen in children with a history of autism or developmental delay, underlying central nervous system disease, and mood disorders. Catatonia is a state of apparent unresponsiveness to external stimuli and can manifest with either negativism, withdrawal and immobility, or with an excited state consisting of impulsivity, nonpurposeful behavior, combativeness, and autonomic instability. Work-up of catatonia should consider medical causes such as infectious or autoimmune encephalitis, nonconvulsive status epilepticus, and other infectious causes. Treatment of catatonia generally consists of benzodiazepines, especially lorazepam, often at high doses and/or frequencies.

Substance use

Substance intoxication or withdrawal can be another source of agitation, often with comorbid altered mental status. Toxicologic work-up can be helpful to elucidate underlying substance ingestion, but often youth are using newer drugs that cannot be picked up on standard testing. Lorazepam is generally recommended for unknown substance use, stimulant intoxication, benzodiazepine or alcohol withdrawal, PCP (phencyclidine) intoxication, or synthetic drugs such as synthetic cannabinoids or cathinones. Haloperidol may be added to these for very severe agitation or comorbid psychosis.

SUMMARY

There are no randomized controlled trials studying psychopharmacologic management of acute agitation in pediatric populations in the ED, or even expert consensus guidelines to direct medication use. At present, an effort is being taken by the authors of this review to obtain national consensus guidelines on the evaluation and management of pediatric acute agitation and aggression using the Delphi method to reach consensus. Research is needed to determine the efficacy of PRN medications and guide clinical decision making. Furthermore, given the increase in patients presenting to the ED for psychiatric complaints, the increased numbers of patients boarding for days in the ED awaiting inpatient beds, and the dearth of child psychiatrists or children's mental health specialists in EDs, an investment in clinical and teaching resources to address this patient population is needed. Child psychiatrists should lead efforts in training emergency medicine physicians and pediatricians, developing nonpharmacologic deescalation protocols, and providing consultation to ED physicians when necessary. Telepsychiatry and other innovative care models may allow child psychiatrists to be available when they cannot be physically present in every ED.

REFERENCES

1. Marzullo LL. Pharmacologic management of the agitated child. Pediatr Emerg Care 2014;30(4):269–75.

2. Dorfman DH, Mehta SD. Restraint use for psychiatric patients in the pediatric emergency department. Pediatr Emerg Care 2006;22:7–12.
3. Lunsky Y, Paquette-Smith M, WEiss JA, et al. Predictors of emergency service use in adolescents and adults with autism spectrum disorder living with family. Emergency Medicine Journal 2015;32(10):787–92.
4. Melese-d'Hospital IA, Olson LM, Cook L, et al. Children presenting to emergency departments with mental health problems. Academic Emergency Medicine 2002; 9:528.
5. Grupp-Phelan J, Harman JS, Kelleher KJ. Trends in mental health and chronic condition visits by children presenting for care at US emergency departments. Public Health Reports 2007;122:55–61.
6. Torio CM, Encinosa W, Berhdahl T, et al. Annaul report on health care for children and youth in the United States: national estimates of cost, utilization and expenditures for children with mental health conditions. Academic Pediatrics 2015;15:19–35.
7. Hilt RJ, Woodward TA, Henderson SW, et al. Agitation treatment for pediatric emergency patients. J Am Acad Child Adolesc Psychiatry 2008;47(2):132–8.
8. Kowalski JM, Kopec KT, Lavelle J, et al. A novel agent for management of agitated delirium: a case series of ketamine utilization in the pediatric emergency department. Pediatric Emergency Care 2017;33(9):e58–62.
9. Cole JB, Moore JC, Nystrom PC, et al. A prospective study of ketamine versus haloperidol for severe prehospital agitation. Clin Toxicol 2016;54(7):556–62.
10. Adimando AA, Poncin YB, Baum CR. Pharmacological management of the agitated pediatric patient. Pediatr Emerg Care 2010;26(11):856–60.
11. Ford M, Delaney KA, Ling L, et al. Clinical Toxicology. Philadelphia: Saunders Press; 2001.
12. Malas N, Brahmbhatt K, McDermott C, et al. Pediatric delirium: evaluation, management and special considerations. Curr Psychiatry Rep 2017;19(9):65.
13. Barzman DH, Brackenbury L, Sonnier L, et al. Brief Rating of Aggression by Children and Adolescents (BRACHA): development of a tool for assessing risk of inpatients' aggressive behavior. J Am Acad Psychiatry Law 2011;39(2):170–9.
14. Connor DF, Melloni RH, Harrison RJ. Overt categorical aggression in referred children and adolescents. J Am Acad Child Adolesc Psychiatry 1998;37:66–73.
15. Pfeffer CR, Solomon G, Plutchik R, et al. Variables that predict assaultiveness in child psychiatric inpatients. J Am Acad Child Psychiatry 1985;24:775–80.
16. Nicholls TL, Ogloff JD, Douglass LLB. Assessing risk for violence among male and female civil psychiatric patients: the HCR-20, PCL: SV, and VSC. Behav Sci Law 2004;22:127–58.
17. Cunningham J, Connor DF, Miller K, et al. Staff survey results and characteristics that predict assault and injury to personnel working in mental health facilities. Aggress Behav 2003;29:31–40.
18. Vivona JM, Ecker B, Halgin R, et al. Self- and other-directed aggression in child and adolescent psychiatric inpatients. J Am Acad Child Adolesc Psychiatry 1995;34:434–44.
19. Tardiff K. The current state of psychiatry in the treatment of violent patients. Arch Gen Psychiatry 1992;49:493–9.
20. Connor DF, Steingard RJ, Cunningham JA, et al. Proactive and reactive aggression in referred child and adolescent. Am J Orthopsychiatry 2004;74:129–36.
21. Cummings MR, Miller BD. Pharmacologic management of behavioral instability in medically ill pediatric patients. Curr Opin Pediatr 2004;16:516–22.
22. Heyneman EK. The aggressive child. Child Adolesc Psychiatr Clin N Am 2003;12: 667–77.

23. McNett M, Sarver W, Wilczewski P. The prevalence, treatment and outcomes of agitation among patients with brain injury admitted to acute care units. Brain Inj 2012;26(9):1155–62.
24. Mossman D. Assessing predictions of violence: being accurate about accuracy. J Consult Clin Psychol 1994;62(4):783–92.
25. Garriga M, Pachiarotti I, Kasper S, et al. Assessment and management of agitation in psychiatry: expert consensus. World J Biol Psychiatry 2016;17(2):86–128.
26. Gaskin CJ, Elsom SJ, Happell B. Interventions for reducing the use of seclusion in psychiatric facilities: review of the literature. Br J Psychiatry 2007;191:298–303.
27. Jayaram G, Samuels J, Konrad SS. Prediction and prevention of aggression and seclusion by early screening and comprehensive seclusion documentation. Innov Clin Neurosci 2012;9(7–8):30–8.
28. Giggie M, Olvera R, Joshi M. Screening for risk factors associated with violence in pediatric patients presenting to a psychiatric emergency department. J Psychiatr Pract 2007;13(4):246–52.
29. Somnier L, Barzman D. Pharmacologic management of acutely agitated pediatric patients. Pediatr Drugs 2011;13(1):1–10.
30. Malas N, Spital L, Fischer J, et al. National survey on pediatric acute agitation and behavioral escalation in academic inpatient pediatric care settings. Psychosomatics 2017;58:299–306.
31. Jonikas JA, Cook JA, Rosen C, et al. A program to reduce use of physical restraint in psychiatric inpatient facilities. Psychiatr Serv 2004;55(7):818–20.
32. Hellerstein DJ, Staub AB. Decreasing the use of restraint and seclusion among psychiatric inpatients. J Psychiatr Pract 2007;13(5):308–17.
33. Meyers J, Schmidt F. Predictive validity of the structured assessment for violence risk in youth (SAVRY) with juvenile offenders. Crim Justice Behav 2008;35:344–55.
34. Ogloff J, Daffern M. The dynamic appraisal of situational aggression: an instrument to assess risk for imminent aggression in psychiatric inpatients. Behav Sci Law 2006;24(6):799–813.
35. Yudofsky SC, Silver JM, Jackson W, et al. The overt aggression scale for the objective rating of verbal and physical aggression. Am J Psychiatry 1986;143(1):35–9.
36. Catapres (clonidine hydrochloride USP). Available at: https://www.accessdata.fda.gov/drugsatfda_docs/label/2012/017407s037lbl.pdf. Accessed January 22, 2018.
37. Strange B. Once daily treatment of ADHD with guanfacine: patient implications. Neuropsychiatr Dis Treat 2008;4(3):499–506.
38. Simons KJ, Watson WTA, Martin TJ, et al. Diphenhydramine: pharmacokinetics and pharmacodynamics in elderly adults, young adults and children. J Clin Pharmacol 1990;30(7):665–71.
39. Simons FER, Simons KJ, Becker AB, et al. Pharmacokinetics and antipruritic effects of hydroxyzine in children with atopic dermatitis. J Pediatr 1984;104(1):123–7.
40. Relling MV, Mulhern RK, Dodge RK, et al. Lorazepam pharmacodynamics and pharmacokinetics in children. J Pediatr 1989;114(4 Pt 1):641–6.
41. Chamberlain JM, Capparelli EV, Brown KM, et al. Pharmacokinetics of intravenous lorazepam in pediatric patients with and without status epilepticus. J Pediatr 2012;160(4):667–72.e2.
42. Holley FO, Magliozzi JR, Stanski DR, et al. Haloperidol kinetics after oral and intravenous doses. Clin Pharmacol Ther 1983;33(4):477–84.

43. Furlanut M, Pierpaola B, Baraldo M, et al. Chlorpromazine disposition in relation to age in children. Clin Pharmacokinet 1990;18(4):329–31.
44. Chlorpromazine. Available at: https://davisplus.fadavis.com/3976/meddeck/pdf/chlorpromazine.pdf. Accessed January 22, 2018.
45. Grothe DR, Calis KA, Jacobsen L, et al. Olanzapine pharmacokinetics in pediatric and adolescent inpatients with childhood-onset schizophrenia. J Clin Psychopharmacol 2000;20(2):220–5.
46. Thyssen A, Vermeulen A, Fuseau E, et al. Population pharmacokinetics of oral risperidone in children, adolescents and adults with psychiatric disorders. Clin Pharmacokinet 2010;49(7):465–78.
47. Sallee FR, Miceli JJ, Tensfeldt T, et al. Single-dose pharmacokinetics and safety of ziprasidone in children and adolescents. J Am Acad Child Adolesc Psychiatry 2006;45(6):720–8.
48. DeVane CL, Nemeroff CB. Clinical pharmacokinetics of quetiapine: an atypical antipsychotic. Clin Pharmacokinet 2001;40(7):509–22.
49. Barry-Walsh J, Daffern M, Duncan S, et al. The prediction of imminent aggression in patients with mental illness and/or intellectual disability using the dynamic appraisal of situational aggression instrument. Australas Psychiatry 2009;17(6):493–6.
50. Daffern M, Howells K. The prediction of imminent aggression and self-harm in personality disordered patients of a high security hospital using the HCR-20 clinical scale and the dynamic appraisal of situational aggression. Int J Forensic Ment Health 2007;6(2):137.
51. Griffith J, Daffern M, Godber T. Examination of the predictive validity of the dynamic appraisal of situational aggression in two mental health units. Int J Ment Health Nurs 2013;22(6):485–92.
52. Lantta T, Kontio R, Daffern M, et al. Using the dynamic appraisal of situational aggression with mental health inpatients: a feasibility study. Patient Prefer Adherence 2016;10:691–701.
53. Barzman D, Mossman D, Sonnier L, et al. Brief Rating of Aggression by Children and Adolescents (BRACHA): a reliability study. J Am Acad Psychiatry Law 2012;40(3):374–82.
54. Silver JM, Yudofsky SC. The overt aggression scale: overview and guiding principles. J Neuropsychiatry Clin Neurosci 1991;3(2):S22–9.
55. Kay SR, Wolkenfelf F, Murrill M. Profiles of aggression among psychiatric patients: I. Nature and prevalence. J Nerv Ment Dis 1988;176:539–46.
56. Halperin J, McKay K, Newcorn J. Development, reliability, and validity of the children's aggression scale-parent version. J Am Acad Child Adolesc Psychiatry 2002;41(3):245–52.
57. Chu CM, Hoo E, Daffern M, et al. Assessing the risk of imminent aggression in institutionalized youth offenders using the dynamic appraisal of situational aggression. J Forens Psychiatry Psychol 2012;2:168–83.
58. Buss AH, Perry M. The aggression questionnaire. J Pers Soc Psychol 1992;63(3):452–9.
59. Buss AH, Warren WL. The aggression questionnaire manual. Los Angeles (CA): Western Psychological Services; 2000.
60. Leckman JF. Rutter's child and adolescent psychiatry. John Wiley; 2017. p. 428–30.
61. Al Sharif S, Ratnapalan S. Managing children with autism spectrum disorder in emergency departments. Pediatr Emerg Care 2016;32(2):101–2.
62. Giarelli E, Nocera R, Turchi R, et al. Sensory stimuli as obstacles to emergency care for children with autism spectrum disorder. Adv Emerg Nurs J 2014;36(2):145–63.

63. Seri S, Pisani F, Thai JN, et al. Pre-attentive auditory sensory processing in autistic spectrum disorder: are electromagnetic measurements telling us a coherent story? Int J Psychophysiol 2007;63:159–63.

64. McGonigle JJ, Venkat A, Beresford C, et al. Management of agitation in individuals with autism spectrum disorders in the emergency department. Child Adolesc Psychiatr Clin N Am 2014;23:83–95.

65. Connor DF, Glatt SJ, Lopez ID, et al. Psychopharmacology and aggression. I: a meta-analysis of stimulant effects on overt/covert aggression-related behaviors in ADHD. J Am Acad Child Adolesc Psychiatry 2002;4:253–61.

66. Aman MG, Bukstein OG, Gadow KD, et al. What does risperidone add to stimulant and parent training for severe aggression in child attention-deficit/hyperactivity disorder? J Am Acad Child Adolesc Psychiatry 2014;53:47–60.e1.

67. Patel BD, Barzman DH. Pharmacology and pharmacogenetics of pediatric ADHD with associated aggression: a review. Psychiatr Q 2013;84:407–15.

68. Storch EA, Arnold EB, Lewis AB, et al. The effect of cognitive behavioral therapy versus treatment as usual for anxiety in children with autism spectrum disorders: a randomized controlled trial. J Am Acad Child Adolesc Psychiatry 2013;52:132–42.e2.

69. Drake J, Johnson N, Stoneck AV, et al. Evaluation of a coping kit for children with challenging behaviors in a pediatric hospital. Pediatr Nurs 2012;38:215–20.

70. Martin A, Krieg H, Esposito F, et al. Reduction of restraint and seclusion through collaborative problem solving: a five-year prospective inpatient study. Psychiatr Serv 2009;59:1406–12.

71. Greene RW, Ablon JS, Martin A. Use of collaborative problem solving to reduce seclusion and restraint in child and adolescent inpatient units. Psychiatr Serv 2006;57:610–2.

72. Busch AB, Shore MF. Seclusion and restraint: a review of recent literature. Harv Rev Psychiatry 2000;8(5):261–70.

73. Wilson MP, Pepper D, Currier GW, et al. The psychopharmacolgy of agitation: consensus statement of the American Association for Emergency Psychiatry Project BETA Psychopharmacology Workgroup. West J Emerg Med 2012;13:26–34.

74. Knox DK, Holloman GH Jr. Use and avoidance of seclusion and restraint: consensus statement of the american association for emergency psychiatry project Beta seclusion and restraint workgroup. Western Journal of Emergency Medicine 2012;13(1):35–40.

75. Vitiello B. P.R.N. medications in child psychiatric patients: a pilot placebo-controlled study. J Clin Psychiatry 1991;52(12):499–501.

76. Vitiello B, Ricciuti AJ, Behar D. PRN medications in child state hospital inpatients. Journal of Clinical Psychiatry 1987;48(9):351–4.

77. Khan SS, Mican LM. A naturalistic evaluation of intramuscular ziprasidone versus intramuscular olanzapine for the management of acute agitation and aggression in children and adolescents. J Child Adolesc Psychopharmacol 2006;16(6):671–7.

78. Jangro WW. Conventional intramuscular sedatives versus ziprasidone for severe agitation in adolescents: case-control study. Child Adolesc Psychiatry Ment Health 2009;3:9.

79. Wolraich MM, Greenhill LL, Pelham W, et al. Randomized, controlled trial of oros methylphenidate once a day in children with attention-deficit/hyperactivity disorder. Pediatrics 2001;108(4):883–92.

80. Pringsheim T, Hirsch L, Gardner D, et al. The pharmacological management of oppositional behaviour, conduct problems, and aggression in children and adolescents with attention-deficit hyperactivity disorder, oppositional defiant

disorder, and conduct disorder: a systematic review and meta-analysis. Part 2: neuroleptics and traditional mood stabilizers. Can J Psychiatry 2015;60(2):52–61.

81. Schieveld JNM, Janssen NJJF. Delirium in the pediatric patient: on the growing awareness of its clinical interdisciplinary importance. JAMA Pediatr 2014; 168(7):595–6.

82. American Psychiatric Association. Diagnostic and statistical manual of mental disorders. 5th edition. Washington, DC: American Psychiatric Publishing; 2013.

83. Cerejeira J, Nogueira V, Luis P, et al. The cholinergic system and inflammation: common pathways in delirium pathophysiology. J Am Geriatr Soc 2012;60: 669–75.

84. Krishnan V, Leung LY, Caplan LR. A neurologist's approach to delirium: diagnosis and management of toxic metabolic encephalopathies. Eur J Intern Med 2013; 25:112–6.

85. Turkel SB, Hanft A. The pharmacologic management of delirium in children and adolescents. Paediatr Drugs 2014;16:267–74.

86. Grover S, Kumar V, Chakrabarti S. Comparative efficacy study of haloperidol, olanzapine, and risperidone in delirium. J Psychosom Res 2011;71:277–81.

87. Sloof VD, Spaans E, van Puijenbroek E, et al. Adverse events of haloperidol for the treatment of delirium in critically ill children. Intensive Care Med 2014;40: 1602–3.

88. Joyce C, Witcher R, Herrup E, et al. Evaluation of the safety of quetiapine in treating delirium in critically ill children: a retrospective review. J Child Adolesc Psychopharmacol 2015;25(9):666–70.

Suicide Evaluation in the Pediatric Emergency Setting

Adrian Jacques H. Ambrose, MD*, Laura M. Prager, MD

KEYWORDS

- Pediatric suicide • Adolescent suicide • Screening tools • Suicide evaluation
- Emergency department setting

KEY POINTS

- Suicide is 1 of the top 3 leading causes of death in the pediatric population and a serious public health concern.
- There are evidence-based screening tools for suicide in the pediatric population; however, predicting suicide risks can be a difficult task.
- The emergency department is an essential source of mental health care for children and adolescents.
- The emergency department may serve as an important opportunity for suicide screening and subsequent targeted interventions and resource management.
- More research is needed in emergency department-based screening algorithms and evidence-driven interventions in the pediatric population.

INTRODUCTION

Suicide has consistently been 1 of the top 3 leading causes of death for youth between 10 and 24 year old since 2008. In young adults between 15 and 24 years old, suicide was the second leading cause of death from 2011 to 2015.[1] In addition, suicide rates have been increasing in this age group in both rural and urban settings.[2] According to the national Youth Risk Behavior Survey, high school students have been reporting significantly higher percentages of high risk suicidal behaviors since 2009, with nearly 1 in 4 female high school students reporting in 2015 that they "seriously considered attempting suicide" within the past year.[3]

Disclosure Statement: Dr A.J.H. Ambrose has no relevant direct financial interest in subject matter or materials discussed in article or with a company making a competing product. L.M. Prager has no relevant direct financial interest in subject matter or materials discussed in article or with a company making a competing product.
Department of Psychiatry, Division of Child and Adolescent Psychiatry, Harvard Medical School, Massachusetts General Hospital, Suite 6A, 55 Fruit Street, Boston, MA 02114, USA
* Corresponding author.
E-mail address: Adrian.Ambrose@mgh.harvard.edu

Abbreviations	
ED	Emergency department
EM	Emergency medicine

The emergency department (ED) often serves as a crucial site of care—to identify risk factors, provide interventions, and facilitate further treatment—for individuals with a high risk of self-harm. In adults aged 18 and older, the rate of ED visits relating to suicidal ideation has been steadily increasing since 2006; in 2013, approximately 1% of all ED visits were due to suicidal ideation.[4] Compared with other age groups presenting to the ED with suicidal ideation, youths were mostly likely to present concurrently with self-inflicted injuries (7.6% for males; 11.1% for females).[4] However, suicidal ideation or other mental health issues may not be the chief complaint and may not be disclosed during an ED visit. One study estimated that only 3% of patients who later reported suicidal ideation specifically indicated mental health chief complaints on their initial ED visit.[5] Parents or guardians are often not aware of their adolescent's mental health needs and high-risk behaviors, including nonlethal self-injuries and suicidal attempts and, therefore, may also fail to share this information with providers.[6–8]

Although most mental health problems diagnosed in adulthood begin in adolescence, a significant portion of these youths do not receive mental health care.[9] In 3 large national surveys, only one-fifth of youths aged 6 to 17 years old who were screened to need mental health services actually received mental health care.[10,11] However, because more than one-third of individuals 16 years and older who completed suicide presented to the ED in the preceding year, EDs seem like an ideal setting to screen young people for suicide risk.[12] A recent study demonstrated that screening pediatric patients in ED setting was acceptable to parents and did not significantly change the duration of stay in the ED.[13] Therefore, screening all pediatric patients, regardless of presenting complaints, for suicide risk in the ED setting may lead to better identification of and more timely intervention for this "hidden" high-risk cohort of patients.

SUICIDE SCREENING IN THE EMERGENCY DEPARTMENT

Given that the ED can be the primary source of health care for more than a million adolescents nationwide, emergency medicine (EM) staff, especially pediatricians who are likely to be the first point of contact, should consider screening for suicide risk during their initial evaluation.[14] Nevertheless, 1 study found that EM clinicians rarely screen for mental illness and, when they do, they base their questions on their own instincts rather than on evidence-based methods. In this study, respondents indicated that the greatest obstacle to mental health screening was time, followed by a lack of an appropriate screening tool.[15] Furthermore, the concept of suicide risk screening for adolescent patients who present to EDs with any complaints (ie, universal screening) remains under debate. Although the Joint Commission on Accreditation of Healthcare Organizations guidelines mandate suicide screening for patients in psychiatric EDs, and for all patients who present with a psychiatric chief complaint (ie, targeted screening) surprisingly, no such mandate exists for EM staff to screen adolescents who present with medical complaints alone.[16] In fact, the US Preventive Services Task Force published guidelines emphasizing that the evidence base is not sufficient either to justify or to support the need for universal suicide screening in this population.[17] Of note, the US Preventive Services Task Force recently recommended universal screening in children and adolescents for depression, which is a common risk factor for suicide.[18]

Despite there being no consistent recommendations for universal screening, there are quite a number of screening tools (**Tables 1** and **2**) designed to help pediatricians and other providers (whether they work in an ED or an outpatient setting) ask questions about suicide risk. For the emergency setting, a few tools, such as, the Ask Suicide Screening Questions and the Risk of Suicide Questionnaire, have been validated in children's hospital EDs.[19–21] Unfortunately, none of these scales has been validated within a general hospital population nor studied prospectively.

Table 1
Common self-administered screening tools for suicidality in youths

Self-Administered Tools	Target Population	Length	Validation
Columbia Health Screen	9th-12th grade students	14 items	Validated with high school students from the general population at school[22]
Suicidal Ideation Questionnaire (SIQ)	15–18 y old 12–14 y old (JR version)	30 items 15 items (JR Version)	Outpatient pediatric/medical setting[21]
Suicide Behaviors Questionnaire (SBQ)	Adapted for adolescents <10 y old (SBQ-C Version)	14 items 4 items (Revised Version) 4 Items (Children Version)	Tested with psychiatric inpatient adolescents and adults, and general high school and college students[23]
Ask-Suicide Screening Questionnaire (ASQ)	10–21 y old	4 items	Validated in ED youths with psychiatric and medical problems[19]
Suicide Probability Scale (SBS)	>14 y old	36 items	Standardized with adolescent and adults from general population, and inpatient college students and adult population[24,25]
Beck Scale for Suicide Ideation (BSSI)	Adolescents	21 items	Development samples included inpatient and outpatient adolescents and adults[26]
Self-harm Behavior Questionnaire (SHBQ)	High school to college-aged students	22 items	Tested with general high school and college students[27,28]
Suicide Ideation Scale (SIS)	College-aged students	10 items	Development samples included general college students[29]
Universal Adolescent Suicide Screening	Adolescents	2 items	Tested in pediatric urgent care center[30]
Risk of Suicide Questionnaire (RSQ)	8–21 y old	4 items	Initially tested in youths with psychiatric symptoms in ED; later expanded to all populations in pediatric ED[31]

Abbreviation: ED, emergency department.

Table 2
Common clinician-administered screening tools for suicidality in youths

Clinician-Administered Tools	Target Population	Length	Validation
Columbia–Suicide Severity Rating Scale (CSSRS)	>10 y old	3–6 items (Screening Versions)	Validated in multiple settings, such as, ED, outpatient, integrated primary care, and inpatient pediatric patients with mental health problems[32–34]
Suicidal Ideation Screening Questionnaire	Adults (including college-aged patients)	4 items	Studied in adult and general medical settings[35]
Home, Education, Activities and peers, Drugs and alcohol, Suicidality, Emotions and behaviors, Discharge resources (HEADS-ED)	4–17 y old	7 items	Developed with youths presenting in the ED with mental health concerns[36]

Abbreviation: ED, emergency department.

RISK FACTOR EVALUATION

Given no clear guidelines or mandate, coupled with a lack of education and provider discomfort (eg, erroneous beliefs that asking about suicide is "putting ideas in an adolescent's head," not being comfortable about how to and what questions to ask), few EM clinicians choose to implement universal suicide screening. In general, EM clinicians consider assessing risk for suicide in a targeted fashion—only in those patients who present with a chief complaint that warrants further mental health evaluation. Once an EM clinician identifies such a patient, he or she generally immediately establishes safety precautions, which may vary depending on individual hospital guidelines and state regulations. These precautions may range from calling for a sitter to stay with the patient and/or signing a commitment paper that allows the hospital to prevent the patient from leaving until the evaluation is completed and an appropriate disposition is determined. Such patients are typically referred for further evaluation by a behavioral health clinician who could be a psychiatrist, psychologist, or social worker, depending on the ED's staffing model.

A comprehensive safety evaluation includes a full history from the patient and collateral sources of information such as parents, other caregivers (outpatient pediatrician or mental health providers), and teachers. Adolescents may try to minimize their safety risk and fail to mention, for example, that they have been texting suicidal statements to friends. A clinician may only learn about such behaviors when he or she talks with the student's guidance counselor, who may have heard this from other students in the school.

The assessment of suicide risk is an imperfect task. Most commonly, evaluators look for risk factors (**Table 3**) and protective factors, and weigh them in ascertaining the likelihood for suicide completion.[37–68] However, predicting suicide behaviors, regardless of the evaluator's skills, can be immensely difficult. A large metaanalysis of longitudinal cohort studies in the psychiatric adult patients in the past 40 years corroborated the challenges in predicting suicide completion.[37] The metaanalysis revealed that at least one-half of all completed suicides actually occurred in the lower

Table 3
Risk factor evaluation for suicidality in youth

Risk Factors	Descriptions
Suicidal ideation	As a core tenet for many psychometrics and screening tools for suicidality, the endorsement of current suicidal ideation often signals a higher risk of subsequent suicidal behaviors.[37–41]
Suicidal attempts	In numerous studies, past suicidal attempts significantly increased the rates of future suicide-related behaviors and suicide completion in outpatient, inpatient, or ED setting.[37,38,44–46]
Acute and chronic stressors	Among pediatric ED patients screening positive for suicidality, approximately 80% reported a presence of a recent life stressor, such as, interpersonal relationships, school-related stressors, health of self/friends/family, witness/victim of violence, and bullying.[47]
Access to lethal methods	The most common methods of completed suicide seemed to be suffocation/hanging, firearms, and overdose/poisoning.[32,40–42,44,48] Hanging/suffocation seemed to be more common in younger children (<12 y old) and females. The use of firearms for suicide completion was more common in males.
Gender	Deaths by suicide in youths are significantly more common in males.[44] In addition, males were more likely to screen positive for suicidality while presenting to the ED with non–suicide-related complaints.[49]
Genetics of suicide (eg, family history)	There may be a genetic component to suicide-related behaviors. Monozygotic twin studies showed significantly greater risk of suicide-related behaviors in comparison with the general population.[50,51] A family history of suicide also seemed to convey greater risks of suicide-related behaviors in youths.[52,53]
Psychiatric history/ recent hospitalization	Among youths with suicidal ideation, an estimated 89.3% would meet criteria for a DSM-IV diagnosis. Similarly, 96.1% of adolescents with at least one suicide attempt would meet criteria for a DSM-IV diagnosis.[54] Of note, a study looking at pediatric suicide completions over almost a decade found that 60% of completed suicides had no report of mental illness or substance abuse.[53]
Substance abuse	In adolescents, alcohol or substance abuse was associated with more depressive symptoms, severe suicidal ideation, recent suicide attempt, and suicide completion.[48,55,56] Another study suggested that adolescents with substance misuse were more than significantly more likely to engage in subsequent suicide-related behaviors.[57]
Interpersonal violence (eg, a victim of physical/sexual abuse, bullying)	History of maltreatment also increases the risk of completed suicide.[43] Bullying seems to be significantly associated with increased rates of mood symptoms and suicide-related behaviors in adolescents.[58,59] One study found that more than three-fourths of adolescents presenting in the ED reported a history of being bullied.[60] In this study, adolescents with a history of cyberbullying were 11.5 times more likely to report suicidal ideation in comparison with adolescents without any bullying.
Intrapersonal violence/NSSI	A longitudinal study estimated that 10% of adolescents will engage in NSSI at least once before the age of 15.[61] Specific characteristics of NSSI including high frequency, duration of 1 year or greater, multiple methods of NSSI, concealment of the NSSI, and severe physical damage caused by NSSI.[62]
Physical illness	Chronic physical illnesses in youths are associated with a slight increase in NSSI, suicidal ideation, and suicidal attempts.[63]

(continued on next page)

Table 3 (continued)	
Risk Factors	**Descriptions**
Social relationships	Conflicts with parents or loss of a parent increased the risks of completed suicide in prepubescent children.[43,64,65] In adolescents with completed suicides, romantic and peer conflicts were more common.[41,54,56]
Special populations	LGBTQ youths reported significantly higher rates of mood symptoms, suicidal ideation, suicidal attempt, and higher severity of suicidality.[66,67] One study found that 22.8% of sexual minority youths attempted suicide in comparison with the 6.6% of heterosexual youths. Of note, Latino, Native American, and Pacific Islander sexual minorities had higher prevalence of suicide attempts in comparison to their White sexual minority counterparts.[68] In general, ethnic minorities, such as African American children, seemed to have disproportionately higher rates of suicide-related behaviors and suicide completions.[43]

Abbreviations: DSM-IV, *Diagnostic and Statistical Manual of Mental Disorders, fourth edition;* ED, emergency department; LGBTQ, lesbian, gay, bisexual, transgender, and queer; NSSI, nonsuicidal self-injury.

risk groups, which were categorized based on each cohort study's individual criteria of risk factors, and only 5% of those in higher risk groups subsequently completed suicides. Similarly, another recent metaanalysis of longitudinal risk factor studies in the past 50 years for both adult and pediatric populations reiterated the limitations in our current risk assessment of suicide.[38] The overall risk factor analysis of these 365 studies suggested that existing risk assessments are relatively weak and potentially inaccurate predictors of suicidal ideation, attempts, and deaths. On a population level, the study noted that the combined risk factor effects might not represent clinically significant effects (ie, 1-year odds of suicide death from 0.013 to 0.019 per 100 people, suicide attempt from 0.33 to 0.49 per 100 people, and suicide ideation from 2 to 3 per 100 people). Despite numerous limitations for generalizability to these metaanalyses, such as the difficulty in determining the impact of the interventions on the higher risk groups, the limited available evidences in evaluating risk factors over hyperacute stages (eg, within hours or days) and limited studies in the pediatric population; both studies clearly underscore the need for a more accurate risk assessment model. Moreover, despite the high prevalence of suicide-related morbidities and mortalities, there is a general dearth of research specifically in the pediatric population. Nevertheless, given the currently limited available of methodology in comprehensive and accurate risk assessment, evaluators continue to focus on the significant risk factors noted herein and use their best clinical judgment.

Overall, the evaluation of risk factors has become increasingly more homogenous over time.[17,37,39–42] In assessing the current risk for the patient, it will be important to consider how each risk factor may affect the short-, intermediate-, and/or long-term risk of suicide. In addition, the presenting complaints (eg, mood symptoms, suicidal ideation, suicidal attempt) may also affect the prioritization of risk factors and, ultimately, disposition.[37–39,41] For example, prior suicidal ideation, hopelessness, a mood disorder (eg, depression, anxiety), and a history of physical or sexual abuse seemed to be better predictors of subsequent suicidal ideation. However, for subsequent suicidal attempts, prior nonsuicidal self-injury, prior suicidal attempt, any kind of personality disorder, and prior psychiatric hospitalization may be better predictive risk factors.[38,40,41,43] As stated, risk factor evaluation is meant to be a general framework to guide interventions and disposition planning. In the pediatric population, it is also essential to consider the specific developmental stage of the child, which may change the relevant risk factors and dictate appropriate disposition resources. In addition, pediatric patients require involvement of parents and guardians, and often have less capacity for self-regulation and a more limited tool-kit of coping skills.

RECOMMENDATIONS AND FUTURE DIRECTIONS
Increasing the Availability of Mental Health Screening in the Emergency Department and Other Nonpsychiatric Settings

A study from an inner-city ED found that, despite youths self-reporting suicidal ideation on screening questions at presentation, only one-fourth of the patient cohort was found to have any additional documentation regarding mental health issues in the electronic medical record and only one-tenth received a psychiatric referral, suggesting a significant missed opportunity for identification and treatment.[5] Furthermore, as noted, almost one-half of pediatric EM clinicians reported that mental health screening is only completed if the patient has a psychiatric chief complaint.[15] Further education of EM clinicians about the need for and potential benefit of universal suicide screening for the child and adolescent population, including appropriate documentation of that assessment in the medical record, is sorely needed.

Across all age groups, almost one-half of individuals (45%) who subsequently complete suicide visited their primary care provider within 1 month before their death.[69] Therefore, implementing a brief suicide screening questionnaire in nonurgent and nonpsychiatric clinician settings, such as a pediatrician's office, may further assist in the identification of high-risk youths.

More Research on Innovative Emergency Department-Based Assessments and Interventions

As stated, the current model of risk assessment may not accurately predict suicide-related behaviors in youths.[38] Current innovations on algorithmic assessment of risks, such as machine learning approaches or natural language processing, which can model highly complex relationships with hundreds of variables, may someday help us to understand the equally intricate nature of suicidal behaviors.[70–72] For example, machine learning approaches with longitudinal health data were able to predict suicidal behaviors with 90% to 95% specificity; similarly, using regression trees and penalized regressions trained with a large US active duty soldier database, a study was able to stratify high risk-groups for the prediction of suicidal behaviors.[73,74]

Because the ED often serves as the entry portal of care for many at-risk youths, ED-based interventions with high-risk youth offers a valuable opportunity for care. A recent large-scale prospective study in adults with recent suicidal attempts or suicidal ideation demonstrated that brief interventions during and after ED visits, which included universal screening and targeted interventions (eg, risk screening by the ED physician, discharge resources, and post-ED telephone call) significantly decreased subsequent suicidal behaviors.[75] Additional research in the pediatric population is needed to assess and stratify risk factors for suicide to allow EM clinicians to provide prompt and appropriate intervention in the ED setting.

REFERENCES

1. Centers for Disease Control and Prevention. 10 leading causes of death. 2016. Available at: https://www.cdc.gov/injury/wisqars/facts.html. Accessed December 23, 2017.
2. Ivey-Stephenson AZ, Crosby AE, Jack SPD, et al. Suicide trends among and within urbanization levels by sex, race/ethnicity, age group, and mechanism of death—United States, 2001–2015. MMWR Surveill Summ 2017;66:1–16.
3. Kann L, McManus T, Harris WA, et al. Youth risk behavior surveillance—United States, 2015. MMWR Surveill Summ 2016;65:1–174.
4. Owens P, Fingar K, Heslin K, et al. Emergency department visits related to suicidal ideation, 2006-2013. Rockville (MD): Agency for Healthcare Research and Quality; 2017. Available at: https://www.hcup-us.ahrq.gov/reports/statbriefs/sb220-Suicidal-Ideation-ED-Visits.jsp.
5. Kemball RS, Gasgarth R, Johnson B, et al. Unrecognized suicidal ideation in ED patients: are we missing an opportunity? Am J Emerg Med 2008;26(6):701–5.
6. Walker M, Moreau D, Weissman MM. Parents' awareness of children's suicide attempts. Am J Psychiatry 1990;147(10):1364–6.
7. Zimmerman JK, Asnis GM. Parents' knowledge of children's suicide attempts. Am J Psychiatry 1991;148(8):1091–2.
8. Young TL, Zimmerman R. Clueless: parental knowledge of risk behaviors of middle school students. Arch Pediatr Adolesc Med 1998;152(11):1137–9.
9. Kessler RC, Berglund P, Demler O, et al. Lifetime prevalence and age-of-onset distributions of DSM-IV disorders in the national comorbidity survey replication. Arch Gen Psychiatry 2005;62(6):593–602.
10. Kataoka SH, Zhang L, Wells KB. Unmet need for mental health care among U.S. children: variation by ethnicity and insurance status. Am J Psychiatry 2002; 159(9):1548–55.
11. Knopf D, Park MJ, Mulye TP. The mental health of adolescents: a national profile, 2008. San Francisco (CA): National Adolescent Health Information Center; 2008.
12. Gairin I, House A, Owens D. Attendance at the accident and emergency department in the year before suicide: retrospective study. Br J Psychiatry 2003;183: 28–33.
13. Horowitz L, Ballard E, Teach SJ, et al. Feasibility of screening patients with nonpsychiatric complaints for suicide risk in a pediatric emergency department: a good time to talk? Pediatr Emerg Care 2010;26(11):787–92.
14. Horowitz LM, Bridge JA, Pao M, et al. Screening youth for suicide risk in medical settings: time to ask questions. Am J Prev Med 2014;47(3 Supplement 2):S170–5.
15. Habis A, Tall L, Smith J, et al. Pediatric emergency medicine physicians' current practices and beliefs regarding mental health screening. Pediatr Emerg Care 2007;23(6):387–93.
16. The Joint Commission. Detecting and treating suicide ideation in all settings. 2016. Available at: https://www.jointcommission.org/assets/1/18/SEA_56_Suicide.pdf. Accessed December 23, 2017.
17. LeFevre ML, U.S. Preventive Services Task Force. Screening for suicide risk in adolescents, adults, and older adults in primary care: U.S. preventive services task force recommendation statement. Ann Intern Med 2014;160(10):719–26.
18. Siu AL, US Preventive Services Task Force. Screening for depression in children and adolescents: US preventive services task force recommendation statement. Pediatrics 2016;137(3):e20154467.

19. Horowitz LM, Bridge JA, Teach SJ, et al. Ask Suicide-Screening Questions (ASQ): a brief instrument for the pediatric emergency department. Arch Pediatr Adolesc Med 2012;166:1–7.

20. Horowitz LM, Wang PS, Koocher GP, et al. Detecting suicide risk in a pediatric emergency department: development of a brief screening tool. Pediatrics 2001;107(5):1133–7.

21. Wintersteen MB. Standardized screening for suicidal adolescents in primary care. Pediatrics 2010;125(5):938–44.

22. Scott M, Wilcox H, Huo Y, et al. School-based screening for suicide risk: balancing costs and benefits. Am J Public Health 2010;100(9):1648–52.

23. Osman A, Bagge CL, Gutierrez PM, et al. The Suicidal Behaviors Questionnaire-Revised (SBQ-R):validation with clinical and nonclinical samples. Assessment 2001;8(4):443–54.

24. Tatman SM, Greene AL, Karr LC. Use of the Suicide Probability Scale (SPS) with adolescents. Suicide Life Threat Behav 1993;23(3):188–203.

25. Eltz M, Evans AS, Celio M, et al. Suicide Probability Scale and its utility with adolescent psychiatric patients. Child Psychiatry Hum Dev 2007;38(1):17–29.

26. Holi MM, Pelkonen M, Karlsson L, et al. Psychometric properties and clinical utility of the Scale for Suicidal Ideation (SSI) in adolescents. BMC Psychiatry 2005;5:8.

27. Gutierrez PM, Osman A, Barrios FX, et al. Development and initial validation of the self-harm behavior questionnaire. J Pers Assess 2001;77(3):475–90.

28. Muehlenkamp JJ, Cowles ML, Gutierrez PM. Validity of the self-harm behavior questionnaire with diverse adolescents. J Psychopathol Behav Assess 2010; 32(2):236–45.

29. Rudd MD. The prevalence of suicidal ideation among college students. Suicide Life Threat Behav 1989;19(2):173–83.

30. Patel A, Watts C, Shiddell S, et al. Universal adolescent suicide screening in a pediatric urgent care center. Arch Suicide Res 2017;1–10. https://doi.org/10.1080/13811118.2017.1304303.

31. Folse VN, Eich KN, Hall AM, et al. Detecting suicide risk in adolescents and adults in an emergency department: a pilot study. J Psychosoc Nurs Ment Health Serv 2006;44(3):22–9.

32. Scott M, Underwood M, Lamis DA. Suicide and related-behavior among youth involved in the juvenile justice system. Child Adolesc Soc Work J 2015;32(6): 517–27.

33. Posner K, Brown GK, Stanley B, et al. The Columbia–Suicide Severity Rating Scale: initial validity and internal consistency findings from three multisite studies with adolescents and adults. Am J Psychiatry 2011;168(12):1266–77.

34. Gipson PY, Agarwala P, Opperman KJ, et al. Columbia-Suicide Severity Rating Scale: predictive validity with adolescent psychiatric emergency patients. Pediatr Emerg Care 2015;31(2):88–94.

35. Cooper-Patrick L, Crum RM, Ford DE. Identifying suicidal ideation in general medical patients. JAMA 1994;272(22):1757–62.

36. Cappelli M, Gray C, Zemek R, et al. The HEADS-ED: a rapid mental health screening tool for pediatric patients in the emergency department. Pediatrics 2012;130(2):e321–7.

37. Large M, Kaneson M, Myles N, et al. Meta-analysis of longitudinal cohort studies of suicide risk assessment among psychiatric patients: heterogeneity in results and lack of improvement over time. PLoS One 2016;11(6):e0156322. DeLuca V, editor.

38. Franklin JC, Ribeiro JD, Fox KR, et al. Risk factors for suicidal thoughts and behaviors: a meta-analysis of 50 years of research. Psychol Bull 2017;143(2):187–232.

39. Eneroth M, Gustafsson Sendén M, Løvseth LT, et al. A comparison of risk and protective factors related to suicide ideation among residents and specialists in academic medicine. BMC Public Health 2014;14:271.

40. Chan MKY, Bhatti H, Meader N, et al. Predicting suicide following self-harm: systematic review of risk factors and risk scales. Br J Psychiatry 2016;209(4):277–83.

41. Hedeland RL, Teilmann G, Jørgensen MH, et al, Study-Associated Pediatric Departments. Risk factors and characteristics of suicide attempts among 381 suicidal adolescents. Acta Paediatr 2016;105(10):1231–8.

42. Steele IH, Thrower N, Noroian P, et al. Understanding suicide across the lifespan: a United States perspective of suicide risk factors, assessment & management. J Forensic Sci 2018. https://doi.org/10.1111/1556-4029.13519.

43. Dykstra HK. Suicide in prepubescent children in the United States: a descriptive analysis of major characteristics and risk factors. Int J Epidemiol 2015; 44(suppl_1):i285–6.

44. Keeshin BR, Gray D, Zhang C, et al. Youth suicide deaths: investigation of clinical predictors in a statewide sample. Suicide Life Threat Behav 2017. https://doi.org/10.1111/sltb.12386.

45. Kene P, Hovey JD. Predictors of suicide attempt status: acquired capability, ideation, and reasons. Psychiatr Q 2014;85(4):427–37.

46. Wang Y, Bhaskaran J, Sareen J, et al. Predictors of future suicide attempts among individuals referred to psychiatric services in the emergency department: a longitudinal study. J Nerv Ment Dis 2015;203(7):507–13.

47. Stanley IH, Snyder D, Westen S, et al. Self-reported recent life stressors and risk of suicide in pediatric emergency department patients. Clin Pediatr Emerg Med 2013;14(1):35–40.

48. Bridge JA, Asti L, Horowitz LM, et al. Suicide trends among elementary school–aged children in the United States from 1993 to 2012. JAMA Pediatr 2015;169(7):673–7.

49. Ballard ED, Cwik M, Eck KV, et al. Identification of at-risk youth by suicide screening in a pediatric emergency department. Prev Sci 2017;18(2):174–82.

50. Roy A, Segal NL, Sarchiapone M. Attempted suicide among living co-twins of twin suicide victims. Am J Psychiatry 1995;152(7):1075–6.

51. Voracek M, Loibl LM. Genetics of suicide: a systematic review of twin studies. Wien Klin Wochenschr 2007;119(15–16):463–75.

52. Hawton K, Saunders KEA, O'Connor RC. Self-harm and suicide in adolescents. Lancet 2012;379(9834):2373–82.

53. Trigylidas TE, Reynolds EM, Teshome G, et al. Paediatric suicide in the USA: analysis of the National child death case reporting system. Inj Prev 2016;22(4):268–73.

54. Nock MK, Green JG, Hwang I, et al. Prevalence, correlates and treatment of lifetime suicidal behavior among adolescents: results from the national comorbidity survey replication – adolescent supplement (NCS-A). JAMA Psychiatry 2013; 70(3). https://doi.org/10.1001/2013.jamapsychiatry.55.

55. King CA, O'Mara RM, Hayward CN, et al. Adolescent suicide risk screening in the emergency department. Acad Emerg Med 2009;16(11):1234–41.

56. Shaw D, Fernandes JR, Rao C. Suicide in children and adolescents: a 10-year retrospective review. Am J Forensic Med Pathol 2005;26(4):309–15.

57. King CA, Berona J, Czyz E, et al. Identifying adolescents at highly elevated risk for suicidal behavior in the emergency department. J Child Adolesc Psychopharmacol 2015;25(2):100–8.

58. Messias E, Kindrick K, Castro J. School bullying, cyberbullying, or both: correlates of teen suicidality in the 2011 CDC youth risk behavior survey. Compr Psychiatry 2014;55(5):1063–8.
59. Selkie EM, Fales JL, Moreno MA. Cyberbullying prevalence among US middle and high school–aged adolescents: a systematic review and quality assessment. J Adolesc Health 2016;58(2):125–33.
60. Alavi N, Reshetukha T, Prost E, et al. Relationship between bullying and suicidal behaviour in youth presenting to the emergency department. J Can Acad Child Adolesc Psychiatry 2017;26(2):70–7.
61. Baetens I, Claes L, Onghena P, et al. Non-suicidal self-injury in adolescence: a longitudinal study of the relationship between NSSI, psychological distress and perceived parenting. J Adolesc 2014;37(6):817–26.
62. Grandclerc S, De Labrouhe D, Spodenkiewicz M, et al. Relations between non-suicidal self-injury and suicidal behavior in adolescence: a systematic review. PLoS One 2016;11(4):e0153760. Botbol M, editor.
63. Barnes AJ, Eisenberg ME, Resnick MD. Suicide and self-injury among children and youth with chronic health conditions. Pediatrics 2010;125(5):889–95.
64. Tishler CL, Reiss NS, Rhodes AR. Suicidal behavior in children younger than twelve: a diagnostic challenge for emergency department personnel. Acad Emerg Med 2007;14(9):810–8.
65. Zainum K, Cohen MC. Suicide patterns in children and adolescents: a review from a pediatric institution in England. Forensic Sci Med Pathol 2017;13(2):115–22.
66. Bouris A, Everett BG, Heath RD, et al. Effects of victimization and violence on suicidal ideation and behaviors among sexual minority and heterosexual adolescents. LGBT Health 2015;3(2):153–61.
67. Marshal MP, Dietz LJ, Friedman MS, et al. Suicidality and depression disparities between sexual minority and heterosexual youth: a meta-analytic review. J Adolesc Health 2011;49(2):115–23.
68. Bostwick WB, Meyer I, Aranda F, et al. Mental health and suicidality among racially/ethnically diverse sexual minority youths. Am J Public Health 2014;104(6):1129–36.
69. Luoma JB, Martin CE, Pearson JL. Contact with mental health and primary care providers before suicide: a review of the evidence. Am J Psychiatry 2002;159(6):909–16.
70. Oh J, Yun K, Hwang J-H, et al. Classification of suicide attempts through a machine learning algorithm based on multiple systemic psychiatric scales. Front Psychiatry 2017;8. https://doi.org/10.3389/fpsyt.2017.00192.
71. Pestian JP, Sorter M, Connolly B, et al. A machine learning approach to identifying the thought markers of suicidal subjects: a prospective multicenter trial. Suicide Life Threat Behav 2017;47. https://doi.org/10.1111/sltb.12312.
72. McCoy TH, Castro VM, Roberson AM, et al. Improving prediction of suicide and accidental death after discharge from general hospitals with natural language processing. JAMA Psychiatry 2016;73(10):1064–71.
73. Kessler RC, Warner LCH, Ivany LC, et al. Predicting U.S. army suicides after hospitalizations with psychiatric diagnoses in the army Study To Assess Risk and Resilience in Servicemembers (Army STARRS). JAMA Psychiatry 2015;72(1):49–57.
74. Barak-Corren Y, Castro VM, Javitt S, et al. Predicting suicidal behavior from longitudinal electronic health records. Am J Psychiatry 2016;174(2):154–62.
75. Miller IW, Camargo CA, Arias SA, et al. Suicide prevention in an emergency department population: the ED-SAFE study. JAMA Psychiatry 2017;74(6):563.

Focused Medical Assessment of Pediatric Behavioral Emergencies

Joshua A. Rocker, MD*, Jeffrey Oestreicher, MD

KEYWORDS

- Medical clearance • Anchoring bias • Momentum bias • Child psychiatry
- Adolescent psychiatry • Suicide • Emergency • Psychiatric admission

KEY POINTS

- No uniformly accepted standard of care exists for medical clearance of pediatric patients with psychiatric complaints.
- Few patients in the emergency department present a broader differential than those with an apparent psychiatric chief complaint.
- Relevant history and examination findings should guide subsequent ancillary testing, interventions, and ultimately disposition because emerging data suggest that reflexive screening laboratory tests are of limited utility.
- Providers should remain mindful of anchoring or diagnosis momentum bias when caring for these patients, especially patients with a psychiatric history.

INTRODUCTION

Accounting for approximately 7% of all pediatric emergency department (ED) visits nationally,[1–4] the number of children presenting with psychiatric issues is increasing faster than any other medical emergency.[5] In addition, these visits require more ED resources, have longer lengths of stay, and have high admission and transfer rates.[1] However, despite this large volume of patients, there is no uniformly accepted standard of care on how providers should medically clear behavioral health patients.

The term medical clearance generally implies that the provider has proved that the psychiatric complaint does not have a medical cause. Often the term "organic" is used to denote a medical disorder as opposed to one that is psychiatric. This terminology reflects a dualist mind-body distinction, which may contribute to an already existing stigma and belief that psychiatric illness has no biological origins.

Disclosures: None.
Division of Pediatric Emergency Medicine, Cohen Children's Medical Center of New York, Northwell Health, 269-01 76th Avenue, New Hyde Park, NY 11040, USA
* Corresponding author.
E-mail address: JRocker@northwell.edu

Child Adolesc Psychiatric Clin N Am 27 (2018) 399–411
https://doi.org/10.1016/j.chc.2018.02.003
1056-4993/18/© 2018 Elsevier Inc. All rights reserved.
childpsych.theclinics.com

Inherent in the task of medical clearance is an obvious medical and ethical obligation to rule out any medical causes for the psychiatric presentation. However, there are tragic case reports of psychiatric symptoms falsely attributed to a primary psychiatric diagnosis before thorough investigation of medical causes.[6] The common thread in these cases is a provider who anchored to a psychiatric diagnosis too early and did so before ruling out organic medical causes, particularly in children with past psychiatric history in whom it is tempting to attribute a behavioral or cognitive change to the underlying psychiatric disease.[5,7–15]

This article provide a rational, stepwise approach to medical clearance of children and adolescents with psychiatric symptoms. It addresses the diverse differential for these presentations, including those caused by medical illness, psychiatric illness, and psychiatric medications, and then discusses what needs to be included in the medical evaluation, which comprises a detailed and thorough physical as well as relevant diagnostic studies.

DIFFERENTIAL DIAGNOSIS

Few patients in the ED present a broader differential than those with an apparent psychiatric chief complaint. Horowitz and Schreiber[16] found that 150 pediatric patients presenting to an ED with a primary psychiatric chief complaint ultimately represented 21 different diagnoses. This article divides the different presentations into 7 unique categories: a psychiatric emergency, a psychiatric concern, a medical emergency caused by a psychiatric condition, a medical emergency/condition caused by a psychiatric medication, a medical condition appearing like a psychiatric condition, a medical condition caused by a psychiatric condition, and a medical condition occurring concurrently with a psychiatric condition (**Table 1**).

When a provider is confronted with distinguishing medical causes from psychiatric ones, it has been shown that certain factors are more suggestive of a medical cause: new or sudden-onset symptoms or onset of symptoms before the age of 12 years, history of visual or tactile hallucinations (as opposed to auditory), seizures, and negative family psychiatric history.[4]

Table 1 Differential diagnosis categories for an apparent psychiatric chief complaint	
Categories of Different Disorders Encountered	**Examples**
Psychiatric emergency	Suicidality, homicidality, uncontrollable violence
Psychiatric concern	Depression, anxiety, conduct disorder, truancy
Medical emergency caused by a psychiatric condition	Asphyxia, toxic overdose, gunshot wound
Medical emergency/condition caused by a psychiatric medication	Neuroleptic malignant syndrome, serotonin syndrome, lithium toxicity
Medical condition appearing like a psychiatric condition	Anemia, brain tumor, encephalitis, thyroid disease, seizures
Medical condition caused by a psychiatric condition	Lacerations from self-inflicted cutting or punching glass in uncontrolled anger
Medical condition co-occurring with a psychiatric condition	UTI, STI, pregnancy, substance abuse concurrent with psychiatric diagnosis

Abbreviations: STI, sexually transmitted infection; UTI, urinary tract infection.

To delve deeper into the differential for various presentations, this article considers the 4 most common presentations for psychiatric issues in the ED (depression/suicidality, anxiety, behavioral issues/aggression, and psychosis) and lists potential medical disorders for each (**Table 2**).

Differential Diagnosis: Depression/Suicidality

In all age groups, depression may not be the documented chief complaint and may instead present with more somatic symptoms or school and behavior problems.[17] Providers can be easily fooled given that somatic complaints like headache, abdominal pain, and fatigue are commonly the presenting symptoms of both psychiatric and medical diseases. Primary depression should be moved higher on the differential in children with multiple provider visits for persistent or recurrent somatic complaints with no determined cause to date.

In children with depressive symptoms or suicidal behaviors, underlying medical issues that may present with similar symptoms must be ruled out, such as anemia, hypothyroidism, pain syndromes, seizures, obstructive sleep apnea, and drug use/withdrawal. Other medical mimickers include endocrinopathies such as uncontrolled diabetes or hypoglycemia, infections like mononucleosis and human immunodeficiency virus (HIV), or other metabolic abnormalities.[6]

Differential Diagnosis: Anxiety

In children, anxiety may manifest as excessive or uncontrollable worry and commonly presents with physical symptoms such as palpitations, restlessness, gastrointestinal upset, and headache. Although in younger children anxiety may be caused by concern for personal safety or the safety of family members, anxiety in older children and adolescents commonly involves school performance or social interaction. Older children may verbalize feelings of irritability, restlessness, anxiety, panic, or nervousness. In

Table 2		
Differences between neuroleptic malignant syndrome and serotonin syndrome		
	Neuroleptic Malignant Syndrome	**Serotonin Syndrome**
Causative agent	Antipsychotics	Serotonergic agents (antidepressants, dextromethorphan), pain medication (tramadol, meperidine), antibiotics (linezolid), antiemetics (ondansetron, metoclopramide)
Vital signs	Hypertension, tachycardia, tachypnea, hyperthermia	Hypertension, tachycardia, tachypnea, hyperthermia
Examination	Wet mucosa and skin Diaphoresis Muscle rigidity Altered mental status Hyporeflexia Normal pupils Normal bowel sounds	Wet mucosa and skin Diaphoresis Muscle rigidity Altered mental status Hyperreflexia, clonus Dilated pupils Hyperactive bowel sounds
Onset of symptoms	Slow, over days	Acute, within few hours
Treatment	Anticholinergics and bromocriptine	Supportive, cyproheptadine, lorazepam

Data from Sadock BJ, Sadock VA, editors. Kaplan & Sadock's synopsis of psychiatry: behavioral sciences/clinical psychiatry. 9th edition. Philadelphia: Lippincott Williams & Wilkins; 2003.

children with intractable or new or sudden-onset anxiety, medical causes that must be ruled out include hypoglycemia, drug toxicity, and thyroid disease.[6]

Differential Diagnosis: Behavioral Issues/Aggression

In acutely violent, impulsive, or aggressive children, medical causes that must be ruled out include infectious central nervous system (CNS) diseases, like meningitis and encephalitis, or structural lesions, including tumors or intracranial bleeding from trauma or arteriovenous malformation. In adolescents, think of intoxication from alcohol or substance abuse with phencyclidine, cocaine, methamphetamine, or anabolic steroids. Rarely, aggression may be the first presentation of metabolic disease like Wilson or late-onset phenylketonuria. Endocrinopathies like thyroid storm or Cushing disease may present as acutely altered mental status with aggressive behavior. After these diseases have been ruled out, primary psychiatric diagnoses like bipolar disorder, psychosis, conduct disorder, oppositional defiant disorder, attention-deficit/hyperactivity disorder, or posttraumatic stress disorder should be considered. It is important to also assess for bullying, victimization, and learning disabilities to help explain the cause of the behavior.[6]

Differential Diagnosis: Psychosis

Psychosis in children may present with hallucinations, delusions, paranoia, acute agitation, confusion, or disorganized behaviors. Psychosis is not a common complaint in pediatrics and may present with the emergence of a range of psychiatric disorders, including schizophrenia, major depressive disorder, bipolar disorder with mania, and schizophreniform disorder. Most of these disorders (schizophrenia, for example) are rare before the age of 13 years, but their incidence increases during adolescence. Because psychosis is uncommon in this age group, it is essential to consider medical causes such as CNS infections, CNS tumors or bleeds, ingestion, or substance abuse, including lysergic acid diethylamide (LSD) cocaine, opioids, barbiturates, and amphetamines, including Ecstasy (3,4-methylenedioxymethamphetamine), all of which may cause hallucinations. When phencyclidine is taken in addition to cannabis, the risk for psychotic symptoms is increased.[18] Auditory hallucinations are more common than visual in psychiatric illness, but can easily be confused with the hallucinations described by a child with pavor nocturnus (night terrors), which occur during sleep more commonly in times of stress or fatigue.[19,20] A host of medical disorders may cause psychotic symptoms, including CNS trauma and infection; intracranial lesions; sepsis; seizures, including interictal or postictal states; diabetic ketoacidosis; and other metabolic disorders.

Differential Diagnosis: Medication Side Effects

Providers should be mindful that many of the medicines commonly used to treat psychiatric disease, including antidepressants, anxiolytics, and antipsychotics, may themselves cause significant side effects or adverse reactions.

Antidepressants

Tricyclic antidepressants (TCAs) have largely been replaced by the newer selective serotonin reuptake inhibitors (SSRIs) given that these newer antidepressants have fewer side effects, including less anticholinergic effects and cardiotoxicity. An important antidepressant side effect, particularly when the antidepressant has been recently initiated, is activation syndrome.[21,22] Symptoms range from agitation and restlessness to disinhibition and aggression to, rarely, psychotic symptoms like hallucinations and delusions.

Benzodiazepines

Commonly given to patients for sedation, paradoxic reactions to benzodiazepines, although rare, are more common in young children and those with developmental disabilities.[23–25] Occurring in less than 1% of patients overall, symptoms are similar to activation syndrome and characterized by increased talkativeness, emotional release, excitement, and excessive movement.

Lithium

With 6850 cases of lithium poisoning documented by the American Association of Poison Control Centers in 2014 and its potential for significant morbidity and mortality, providers should be familiar with the multiple presentations of lithium toxicity.[26] Acute ingestion typically presents with tremors, confusion, lethargy, seizures, and gastrointestinal symptoms. Chronic lithium toxicity, however, may present with signs of hypothyroidism (fatigue, weight gain, constipation, cold intolerance, or increased menstrual flow and cramping in girls and young women) or nephrogenic diabetes insipidus (DI), which may present with new onset of extreme thirst and frequent, dilute urine. Hagino and colleagues[27] found that 60% of aggressive and/or mood-disordered children started on lithium therapy developed 1 or more types of side effects, most commonly CNS effects, and found that they occurred frequently in children aged 6 years and younger during the initiation phase of treatment over the first 2 weeks. Importantly, toxicity has been reported even with normal serum concentrations.[28]

Antipsychotics

All antipsychotic medications have the potential to cause extrapyramidal symptoms (EPS), including dystonic reactions and akathisia. Akathisia, or restlessness and difficulty sitting still, has been reported in up to 10% of pediatric patients on antipsychotics[29] and is the most common form of EPS. Acute dystonic reactions are characterized by the rapid and involuntary contraction of large muscle groups, ultimately presenting as torticollis, retrocollis, or oculogyric crisis.[30,31] Acute dystonic reactions can be distinguished from seizures in general by the maintenance of consciousness in dystonic reactions and their relative responsiveness to diphenhydramine or benztropine.

Neuroleptic Malignant Syndrome and Serotonin Syndrome

Two of the most serious and life-threatening adverse reactions to psychotropic medications are neuroleptic malignant syndrome (NMS) and serotonin syndrome (SS). NMS is rare, occurring in about 0.2% of patients treated with neuroleptics[32] and is reportedly most commonly with dopamine antagonists (atypical antipsychotics, some antiemetics like metoclopramide, and TCAs). It is a clinical diagnosis that may present classically as the tetrad of fever, rigidity, mental status changes, and autonomic instability; however, it more frequently has a variable presentation making it challenging to identify, with potentially serious consequences given its estimated mortality of 20%.[33]

Clinically similar to and often confused with NMS, SS or serotonin toxicity presents classically with the triad of acute mental status change, autonomic hyperactivity, and neurologic signs like myoclonus. In actuality, SS presents as a clinical spectrum ranging from benign gastrointestinal upset to life-threatening rhabdomyolysis, seizures, and autonomic instability. The differentiation between NMS and SS is especially difficult given that SS may also cause hyperthermia, hypertension, and muscle rigidity (see **Table 2**).[34]

More often implicated in SS are the SSRIs,[35,36] especially when more than 1 agent is being taken. Other medications in conjunction with an SSRI have been implicated as causative agents in SS, including over-the-counter cough and cold medications containing dextromethorphan, certain pain medications (tramadol, meperidine), antibiotics (linezolid), antiemetics (ondansetron, metoclopramide), drugs of abuse (MDMA [3,4-methylenedioxy-methamphetamine], cocaine), and dietary supplements (St John's wort, ginseng).[37–40]

MEDICAL EVALUATION

The approach to a child or adolescent presenting with a psychiatric complaint should be as methodical as for one with a medical complaint. That is, the ABCs (airway, breathing, circulation) are paramount and the patient's presenting symptoms, relevant history, and examination findings should guide subsequent ancillary testing, consultations, interventions, and ultimately disposition. Patients with new-onset symptoms should be assumed to have an underlying medical cause until proved otherwise because new-onset psychiatric disease is an exclusionary diagnosis.

Thorough evaluation, including review of systems, must uncover those physical complaints that may point to a medical diagnosis; for example, vomiting, weakness, visual or gait/balance changes, or dysuria. If the patient endorses suicidality, the provider should evaluate the degree of concern (see Adrian Jacques H. Ambrose and Laura M. Prager's article, "Suicide Evaluation in the Pediatric Emergency Setting," in this issue). Inquire about previous medical or psychiatric diagnoses and whether medications are prescribed, whether the patient or parent is compliant. It is important to inquire about sexual orientation/history, possible sexually transmitted infections, or pregnancy. **Box 1** provides an overall approach to the evaluation of patients presenting with psychiatric complaints.

Box 1
Stepwise approach to evaluation

- History of present illness: description of present problems and symptoms
- Information about health, illness and treatment (both physical and psychiatric), including current medications
- Parent and family health and psychiatric histories
- Information about the child's development
- Information about the child's experience in school and friends
- Information about family relationships
- Interview of the child
- Interview of parents/guardians
- Physical examination of child
- Mental status examination of child
- If needed, laboratory studies such as blood tests, radiographs, or special assessments (eg, psychological, educational, speech and language evaluation)

Any medical disorder revealed during evaluation, whether or not it is contributing to the patient's acute presentation, should be stabilized and treated (urinary tract infection or deep lacerations, for example), so that the patient's psychiatric symptoms may then safely be addressed. Completion of the medical clearance evaluation indicates to all interdisciplinary teams that any medical issues have been treated and/or ruled out and the patient may now safely undergo psychiatric consultation.

Physical Examination

The evaluation of a patient with a psychiatric complaint should always begin with a review of a complete set of vital signs. Unexplained tachycardia (meaning, for example, in a patient without the appearance of pain, anxiety or agitation, fever, or dehydration) needs to be further evaluated; for instance, could this patient's increased heart rate be a subtle finding of hypovolemia in a patient on lithium who now has DI? Hypoventilation may suggest opiate use, whereas hyperventilation may be an indication of acidosis from DKA, a toxic ingestion, or a significant infection. Hypertension in the setting of altered mental status may indicate hypertensive encephalopathy. An increase in the patient's temperature may point to an infectious cause, a toxic overdose, or SS/NMS, whereas hypothermia may suggest barbiturate ingestion or hypoglycemia.

Once the vitals have been vetted, the physical examination should begin with the general appearance and mental state of the child. Establish the patient's baseline mental status. For example, the posture and grooming or whether the patient is alert and oriented or reacting to internal stimuli may reveal important clues to a primary psychiatric emergency. Also be sure that the patient is fully but sensitively exposed (in a gown, for example) in order to not miss subtle evidence of injury (including self-injury or originating from abuse). All patients should undergo careful examination of cardiac, respiratory, and abdominal systems. In addition, thorough examination of the head, neck, and scalp may reveal signs of meningitis (photophobia, nuchal rigidity), trauma, or increased intracranial pressure (papilledema on fundoscopic examination). The thyroid gland should be examined for possible disease, including enlargement or tenderness, which may suggest possible hypothyroidism or hyperthyroidism.

Careful eye examination may suggest a specific toxidrome; for example, pupil dilatation (sympathomimetic or anticholinergic) or constriction (cholinergic or opioid). Bloodshot eyes may point to a lack of sleep or, in the setting of abnormal vital signs, an illicit ingestion like marijuana. Assessing for the quality of patient comfort with eye contact during the examination may also be an important clue to possible behavioral disorder such as social anxiety, autism spectrum disorder, psychosis, or depression. With regard to the extremities, evaluate the skin for self-injurious behaviors like cutting (classic areas are the nondominant forearms, but both should be evaluated as well as inner thighs, shoulders, ankles, stomach). Children with an impulse control disorder, anxiety, or a tic may pick at their skin, pull their hair or eyebrows/lashes, or pathologically bite their nails and cuticles. Children with bulimia may have erythema on the base of their pointer fingers and, on examination of the oropharynx, teeth erosion from frequent self-induced emesis.

Neurologic examination should evaluate for any focal deficits, which certainly heighten a suspicion for medical disorder.[41,42] Assess for any alteration in mental or neurologic status that may suggest an easily correctable hypoglycemia or a potentially life-threatening intracranial bleed from trauma or ruptured arteriovenous malformation. Examine the extremities for muscle tone and weakness, fasciculations or dystonic posturing, impaired coordination, and hyporeflexia or hyperreflexia. Clinicians must distinguish between neurologic and psychiatric findings, because psychiatric symptoms alone may represent primary psychiatric disorder; however, in conjunction with neurologic findings, psychiatric symptoms likely represent a medical emergency.

Diagnostic Evaluation

There are 2 basic practices used by practitioners when performing diagnostic evaluations:

1. Automatic or routine behavioral health screening tests (**Box 2**)
2. Directed screening tests based on history or clinical findings

A consensus report regarding adult behavioral health patients from the American College of Emergency Physicians stated in a 2017 position paper that, "Routine or ancillary laboratory testing for psychiatric patients has little or no use in the ED,"[43] with the caveat that patients with higher rates of disease (eg, elderly, immunosuppressed, new-onset psychosis, substance abuse) may benefit from testing. They based their conclusion on 2 studies that both concluded that laboratory evaluation after medical screening rarely changes management or disposition. Janiak and Schreiber[44] found in 2012 that among 502 consecutive patients admitted to a psychiatric service, all of whom received screening tests, only 1 patient (0.19%) had a test performed that changed management. That same year, Parmar and colleagues[45] found that, in 598 patients presenting to an ED for a psychiatric complaint, among the 44% of patients with laboratory tests, only 1 patient (0.5%) had a laboratory result that changed the patient's disposition. There were abnormal test results in each of these studies but findings of anemia, hyperglycemia, or urine toxicology, for example, were generally anticipated and did not require intervention.[41,44,46]

Although no similar consensus has been published for the pediatric population, similar data, although limited, are emerging. In 2011, Feldman and Chen[47] reviewed 153 sequential pediatric psychiatric admissions and found that although 97.2% of admitted children with screening tests had an abnormal result, only 4 of them (<0.5%: positive urinalysis, abnormal liver function tests, abnormal comprehensive metabolic panel, and increased serum glucose level) changed management or required immediate attention. In 2006, Santiago and colleagues[48] prospectively analyzed 54 pediatric patients' screening tests for medical clearance for psychiatric admission; no patient had an abnormal result that affected management within the

---

Box 2
Laboratory screening tests for medical clearance

- Point of care glucose
- Complete blood count with differential
- Complete metabolic panel
- Thyroid function panel
- Urinalysis, urine pregnancy
- Toxicology screen (urine and serum)
- Sexually transmitted infection panel including HIV and rapid plasma reagin
- Serum levels of any medications, if appropriate

From Sadock BJ, Sadock VA, editors. Kaplan & Sadock's synopsis of psychiatry: behavioral sciences/clinical psychiatry. 9th edition. Philadelphia: Lippincott Williams & Wilkins; 2003; with permission.

ED. Most recently, Donofrio and colleagues[49] retrospectively reviewed 1082 pediatric patients presenting to an academic pediatric ED for medical clearance of an acute psychiatric emergency and concluded that "while patients with screening tests had a significantly longer length or stay, no urine toxicology test, screening blood laboratory test, or urinalysis alone led to a medical admission."[49] The investigators also stated that no patient was found to have an organic cause of the symptoms based on screening tests alone.

Multiple studies have also shown the diagnostic futility of urine drug screens (UDS) in the ED setting.[48–51] Shihabuddin and colleagues[50] in 2013 retrospectively reviewed 539 pediatric patients presenting to the pediatric ED for psychiatric evaluation and found that although 62 had a positive UDS, none led to a documented change in management or medical intervention in the pediatric ED. Given that patient-reported history of drug use strongly correlated with the UDS results, the investigators concluded that, "patient-reported history was sufficient"[50] to guide further diagnostics and medical management, including the decision for medical clearance. Importantly, a negative UDS is not particularly meaningful because many recreational drugs (many of the hallucinogens or synthetic cannabinoids, for example) are not detected on a standard toxicology screen. However, given the current well-publicized opioid epidemic and the well-documented connection between psychiatric illness and illicit drug use, although reflexively obtaining a drug screen is not supported by recent literature, toxicology tests should be obtained if evaluation reveals red flags or history is incomplete.

In summary, although there is no interdisciplinary consensus on ancillary testing for a psychiatric complaint in the pediatric population, the emerging data seem to suggest that reflexive screening tests are of limited utility and, instead, providers should reserve testing for patients with concerning history or suspicious findings on clinical examination. For example, testing for sexually transmitted infections, including HIV, in patients who are engaging in high-risk sexual behavior or intravenous drug use is an example of testing performed because of a concerning history. Performing thyroid studies in a patient whose examination reveals a goiter or whose symptoms are suggestive of thyroid disease (palpitations, heat intolerance, and weight loss suggestive of hyperthyroidism) is an example of testing performed because of a concerning symptom of physical finding.

Providers should also consider more conservative management and possibly a bias toward testing in those patients at higher risk for medical complications; for example, patients with known medical comorbidities, substance abuse, or concurrent medical symptoms. Although there is no standard panel of laboratory tests for medical clearance of patients with psychiatric complaints, **Box 2** outlines the most common tests providers may consider. Toxicology screens and pregnancy tests in women of child-bearing age are the most frequently obtained laboratory tests.[6]

Depending on the clinical scenario, other testing may be indicated, including a chest radiograph, electrocardiogram (ECG), electroencephalogram, head computed tomography or MRI, and lumbar puncture, although none of these tests should be routinely performed. For example, head imaging is warranted for patients with papilledema, which raises suspicion for an intracranial mass or inflammatory neurologic process. It is common practice to obtain head imaging for new-onset visual hallucinations, although there is no pediatric literature to support this. It is important to communicate with the psychiatric provider team about obtaining additional baseline tests, because some facilities request a baseline ECG for QT interval or a set of liver enzymes before starting psychotropic medications. However, if these baseline tests are performed, their results should not hold up an admission or transfer for further psychiatric evaluation if the patient is otherwise medically cleared.

SUMMARY

There is no uniformly accepted definition of medical clearance of pediatric patients with a psychiatric health complaint, nor is there consensus on how to achieve this clearance and what ancillary testing or procedures should be involved. This lack of clarity on what constitutes medical clearance, in conjunction with the vast differential diagnosis outlined earlier, leads to multiple pitfalls while managing these patients. The surest way to not miss the subtle medical disease masquerading as a psychiatric symptom is to perform a thorough history and physical examination on every patient who presents with a psychiatric chief complaint. Although the data support deferring routine screening tests, any red flags uncovered during history and physical examination should prompt a more aggressive work-up. Most importantly, providers must resist the urge to anchor too early to a primary psychiatric diagnosis before thorough evaluation has ruled out a medical cause, because the consequences of being wrong may be devastating.

REFERENCES

1. Larkin GL, Claassen CA, Emond JA, et al. Trends in U.S. emergency department visits for mental health conditions, 1992 to 2001. Psychiatr Serv 2005;56: 671–7.
2. Dolan MA, The Committee on Pediatric Emergency Medicine. Technical report–pediatric and adolescent mental health emergencies in the emergency medical services system. Pediatrics 2011;127:E1356–66.
3. Simon AE, Schoendorf KC. Emergency department visits for mental health conditions among US children, 2001-2011. Clin Pediatr 2014;53(14):1359–66.
4. Baren JM, Mace SE, Hendry PL, et al. Children's mental health emergencies–part 2: emergency department evaluation and treatment of children with mental health disorders. Pediatr Emerg Care 2008;24(7):485–98.
5. Mahajan P, Alpern ER, Grupp-Phelan J, et al. Epidemiology of psychiatric-related visits to emergency departments in a multicenter collaborative research pediatric network. Pediatr Emerg Care 2009;25:715–20.
6. Fleisher GR, Ludwig S, Henretig FM. Textbook of pediatric emergency medicine. 4th edition. Philadelphia: Lippincott Williams & Wilkins; 2000.
7. Zayac A, Grewal S, Hegazy H. Anchors aweigh: the dangers of anchoring bias in a case of serotonin syndrome. Crit Care Med 2016;44(12):541.
8. Croskerry P. From mindless to mindful practice–cognitive bias and clinical decision making. N Engl J Med 2013;368(26):2445–8.
9. Goldstein AB, Horwitz SM. Child and adolescent psychiatric emergencies in nonsuicide-specific samples: the state of the research literature. Pediatr Emerg Care 2006;22(5):379–84.
10. Babu K, Boyer E. Emergency department evaluation of acute onset psychosis in children. Waltham (MA): UpToDate; 2016. Available at: http://www.uptodate.com/contents/emergency-department-evaluation-of-acute-onset-psychosis-in-children.
11. Chun TH, Mace SE, Katz ER. Evaluation and management of children and adolescents with acute mental health or behavioral problems. Part I: common clinical challenges of patients with mental health and/or behavioral emergencies. Pediatrics 2016;138(3) [pii:e20161571].

12. Delirium WM. In: Hales R, Yudofsky S, editors. Textbook of neuropsychiatry. Washington, DC: American Psychiatric Press; 1987. p. 89–106.
13. Shaffer D, Gould MS, Fisher P, et al. Psychiatric diagnosis in child and adolescent suicide. Arch Gen Psychiatry 1996;53(4):339–48.
14. Hauptman AJ, Benjamin S. The differential diagnosis and treatment of catatonia in children and adolescents. Harv Rev Psychiatry 2016;24(6):379–95.
15. Weller E, Weller R, Svadjian H. Mood disorders. In: Lewis M, editor. Child and adolescent psychiatry: a comprehensive textbook. Baltimore (MD): Williams and Wilkins; 1996. p. 650–5.
16. Horowitz LM, Schreiber MD. Psychological factors in emergency medical services for children. An introduction to the bibliography of psychological, behavioral, and medical literature, 1991Y1998. Bibliographies in Psychology 1999;18.
17. Mojica M. PEM guides. New York: NYU Langone Medical Center; 2015. iBooks. Available at: https://itunes.apple.com/WebObjects/MZStore.woa/wa/viewBook?id=1039923332.
18. Edelsohn GA. Hallucinations in children and adolescents: considerations in the emergency setting. Am J Psychiatry 2006;163(5):781–5.
19. Thiedke C. Sleep disorders and sleep problems in childhood. Am Fam Physician 2001;63(2):277–85.
20. Hetrick SE, McKenzie JE, Cox GR, et al. Newer generation antidepressants for depressive disorders in children and adolescents. Cochrane Database Syst Rev 2012;(11):CD004851.
21. Nischal A, Tripathi A, Nischal A, et al. Suicide and antidepressants: what current evidence indicates. Mens Sana Monogr 2012;10(1):33–44.
22. Goodman WK, Murphy TK, Storch EA. Risk of adverse behavioral effects with pediatric use of antidepressants. Psychopharmacology (Berl) 2007;191(1):87–96.
23. Kandemir H, Yumru M, Kul M, et al. Behavioral disinhibition, suicidal ideation, and self-mutilation related to clonazepam. J Child Adolesc Psychopharmacol 2008;18(4):409.
24. Kalachnik JE, Hanzel TE, Sevenich R, et al. Benzodiazepine behavioral side effects: review and implications for individuals with mental retardation. Am J Ment Retard 2002;107(5):376–410.
25. Mancuso CE, Tanzi MG, Gabay M. Paradoxical reactions to benzodiazepines: literature review and treatment options. Pharmacotherapy 2004;24(9):1177–85.
26. Bronstein AC, Spyker DA, Cantilena LR Jr, et al. 2010 annual report of the American Association of Poison Control Centers' National Poison Data System (NPDS): 28th annual report. Clin Toxicol (Phila) 2011;49(10):910–41.
27. Hagino OR, Weller EB, Weller RA, et al. Untoward effects of lithium treatment in children aged four through six years. J Am Acad Child Adolesc Psychiatry 1995;34(12):1584–90.
28. Speirs J, Hirsch SR. Severe lithium toxicity with "normal" serum concentrations. Br Med J 1978;1(6116):815–6.
29. Forcen FE, Radwan K, Arauz A, et al. Drug-induced akathisia in children and adolescents. J Child Adolesc Psychopharmacol 2017;27(1):102–3.
30. Correll CU. Assessing and maximizing the safety and tolerability of antipsychotics used in the treatment of children and adolescents. J Clin Psychiatry 2008;69(Suppl 4):26–36.
31. Owens D. A guide to the extrapyramidal side-effects of antipsychotic drugs. Cambridge (United Kingdom): Cambridge University Press; 2014.

32. Caroff SN, Mann SC. Neuroleptic malignant syndrome. Med Clin North Am 1993; 77(1):185.

33. Bhanushali MJ, Tuite PJ. The evaluation and management of patients with neuroleptic malignant syndrome. Neurol Clin 2004;22:389–411.

34. Chun TH, Mace SE, Katz ER, American Academy of Pediatrics Committee on Pediatric Emergency Medicine, American College of Emergency Physicians Pediatric Emergency Medicine Committee. Evaluation and management of children with acute mental health or behavioral problems. Part II: recognition of clinically challenging mental health related conditions presenting with medical or uncertain symptoms. Pediatrics 2016;138(3) [pii:e20161573].

35. Perry PJ, Wilborn CA. Serotonin syndrome vs neuroleptic malignant syndrome: a contrast of causes, diagnoses, and management. Ann Clin Psychiatry 2012; 24(2):155–62.

36. Bronstein AC, Spyker DA, Cantilena LR Jr, et al. 2011 annual report of the American Association of Poison Control Centers' National Poison Data System (NPDS): 29th annual report. Clin Toxicol (Phila) 2012;50(10):911.

37. Boyer EW, Shannon M. The serotonin syndrome. N Engl J Med 2005;352(11): 1112–20.

38. Huang V, Gortney JS. Risk of serotonin syndrome with concomitant administration of linezolid and serotonin agonists. Pharmacotherapy 2006;26(12):1784–93.

39. Dobry Y, Rice T, Sher L. Ecstasy use and serotonin syndrome: a neglected danger to adolescents and young adults prescribed selective serotonin reuptake inhibitors. Int J Adolesc Med Health 2013;25(3):193–9.

40. Sternbach H. The serotonin syndrome. Am J Psychiatry 1991;148(6):705–13.

41. Korn CS, Currier GW, Henderson SO. "Medical clearance" of psychiatric patients without medical complaints in the emergency department. J Emerg Med 2000; 18(2):173–6.

42. Carney C, Cetan Health Consultants LLC. Medical assessment of the patient with mental symptoms (Merck manual professional version). Indianapolis (IN): MDwise; 2012.

43. American College of Emergency Physicians Clinical Policies Subcommittee on the Adult Psychiatric Patient, Nazarian DJ, Broder JS, Thiessen MEW, et al. Clinical policy: critical issues in the diagnosis and management of the adult psychiatric patient in the Emergency Department. Ann Emerg Med 2017;69(4):480–98.

44. Janiak BD, Atteberry S. Medical clearance of the psychiatric patient in the emergency department. J Emerg Med 2012;43(5):866–70.

45. Parmar P, Goolsby CA, Udompanyanan K, et al. Value of mandatory screening studies in emergency department patients cleared for psychiatric admission. West J Emerg Med 2012;13:388–93.

46. Olshaker JS, Browne B, Jerrard DA, et al. Medical clearance and screening of psychiatric patients in the emergency department. Acad Emerg Med 1997; 4(2):124–8.

47. Feldman L, Chen Y. The utility and financial implications of obtaining routine laboratory screening upon admission for child and adolescent psychiatric inpatients. J Psychiatr Pract 2011;17:375–81.

48. Santiago LI, Tunik MG, Foltin GL, et al. Children requiring psychiatric consultation in the pediatric emergency department: epidemiology, resource utilization, and complications. Pediatr Emerg Care 2006;22(2):85–9.

49. Donofrio JJ, Santillanes G, McCammack BD, et al. Clinical utility of screening laboratory tests in pediatric psychiatric patients presenting to the emergency department for medical clearance. Ann Emerg Med 2014;63(6):666–75.e3.

50. Shihabuddin BS, Hack CM, Sivitz AB. Role of urine drug screening in the medical clearance of pediatric psychiatric patients: is there one? Pediatr Emerg Care 2013;29(8):903–6.
51. Fortu JM, Kim IK, Cooper A, et al. Psychiatric patients in the pediatric emergency department undergoing routine urine toxicology screens for medical clearance: results and use. Pediatr Emerg Care 2009;25(6):387–92.

An Emergency Department Clinical Pathway for Children and Youth with Mental Health Conditions

Mona Jabbour, MD, MEd[a,b],*, Jeffrey Hawkins, MSW[c],
Doreen Day, MHSc[d], Paula Cloutier, MA[e],
Christine Polihronis, PhD[e], Mario Cappelli, PhD[e,f,g],
Allison Kennedy, PhD[h], Clare Gray, MBA, MD[h]

KEYWORDS

- Mental health/addictions • Clinical pathway • Implementation • HEADS-ED
- Screening tools • Emergency department (ED) • Community mental health

KEY POINTS

- Children and youth are increasingly seeking services for mental health/addictions concerns, putting increasing burden on hospital emergency departments.
- Care of children and youth with acute mental health/addiction conditions is fragmented; improved management by standardizing care and facilitating transition between emergency department and outpatient services is needed.

Continued

Disclosure Statement: The authors have no financial or commercial conflicts of interest to disclose.
[a] Division of Emergency Medicine, Department of Pediatrics, Children's Hospital of Eastern Ontario, 401 Smyth Road, Ottawa, Ontario K1H 8L1, Canada; [b] Faculty of Medicine, Department of Pediatrics, University of Ottawa, 401 Smyth Road, Ottawa, Ontario, K1H 8L1, Canada; [c] Hands TheFamilyHelpNetwork.ca, 391 Oak Street East, North Bay, Ontario, P1B 1A3, Canada; [d] The Provincial Council for Maternal and Child Health, 555 University Avenue, Toronto, Ontario M5G 1X8, Canada; [e] Psychiatric and Mental Health Research, Children's Hospital of Eastern Ontario Research Institute, 401 Smyth Road, Ottawa, Ontario K1H 8L1, Canada; [f] Department of Psychiatry, University of Ottawa, 5457-1145 Carling Avenue, Ottawa, Ontario, K1Z 7K4, Canada; [g] Faculty of Graduate and Postdoctoral Studies, School of Psychology, University of Ottawa, 136 Jean-Jacques Lussier, Vanier Hall, Ottawa, Ontario, K1N 6N5, Canada; [h] Mental Health, Children's Hospital of Eastern Ontario, 401 Smyth Road, Ottawa, Ontario K1H 8L1, Canada
* Corresponding author. Division of Emergency Medicine, Department of Pediatrics, Children's Hospital of Eastern Ontario, 401 Smyth Road, Ottawa, Ontario K1H 8L1, Canada.
E-mail address: Jabbour@cheo.on.ca

Child Adolesc Psychiatric Clin N Am 27 (2018) 413–425
https://doi.org/10.1016/j.chc.2018.02.005
childpsych.theclinics.com

Continued

- An emergency department mental health clinical pathway has been developed, disseminated; and implemented in several pilot settings; an implementation toolkit is available online to support local implementation efforts.
- Experiences from these pilots provide valuable lessons for tailoring future implementations.

INTRODUCTION

The hospital emergency department (ED) is an important and frequently accessed entry point for children and youth across North America with mental health and addictions (MH/A) concerns.[1–7] More than 50% of youth seeking MH care use the ED as the first point of contact without previously seeking outpatient MH care[6] and repeat visitors account for a large proportion of presentations with estimates ranging from 12% to 43%.[8] Not only are EDs seeing an increased volume of MH patients,[7,9] the duration of stay for MH visits is up to twice that of other conditions[10] with multiple factors often contributing to longer wait times.[11] Increased duration of stay is also associated with higher costs[12]; consequently, hospital EDs are under great pressure to manage these wait times without sacrificing quality patient care.

In addition to their pivotal role as an access point for MH/A services, hospital EDs also serve as a point of interim care for children and youth awaiting a definitive MH assessment and treatment in hospital or in the community. Many EDs are challenged in managing children and youth with MH/A owing to a lack of clinical resources, standardized screening tools, and/or training.[13,14] This problem is compounded by the lack of reliable, integrated, and streamlined referral processes to appropriate resources in the community. The MH system in Canada and the United States is complex, fragmented, and limited,[15–17] and the transition between emergent care and outpatient care for MH conditions remains problematic.[1] In particular, there is poor understanding among ED and community MH agencies (CMHAs) regarding what services each organization provides. More timely and accessible outpatient services have been recommended to improve this currently problematic transition between acute and outpatient care.

CLINICAL PATHWAYS

A clinical pathway is a tool that operationalizes best evidence and supports quality care delivery within and across interdisciplinary teams into a standardized, accessible, and structured point-of-care format.[18] Because clinical pathways define standardized care processes that can be anticipated by interdisciplinary health teams, many potential benefits have been demonstrated with their use, including improved efficiency, patient safety, and outcomes, as well as decreased hospital costs.[19–27] Clinical pathways are being increasingly used in EDs and recommended by broader health systems internationally as a form of quality improvement.[28,29] Although EDs have embraced clinical pathways to improve the standard practice for specific medical conditions and pediatric behavioral presentations,[30,31] we did not find any published clinical pathways focused on emergency management of overall pediatric MH/A presentations.

The Provincial Council for Maternal Child Health in Ontario convened an interdisciplinary work group to develop an evidence-informed clinical pathway to guide and support the care of children and youth presenting to an ED with MH/A concerns and to integrate follow-up services in relevant CMHAs. This report describes the development of and early implementation experience with this clinical pathway.

DEVELOPMENT OF THE EMERGENCY DEPARTMENT MENTAL HEALTH CLINICAL PATHWAY
Work Group

To ensure appropriate representation of relevant areas of expertise and perspectives, the work group included clinicians, researchers, educators, and administrators, all involved in the care of children, youth, and families. Representatives from the provincial funders for child and youth MH care were also included. The work group co-chairs included a CMHA executive director (J.H.) and a pediatric emergency physician/researcher (M.J.). As shown in **Box 1**, the group's activities were guided by clear terms of reference with the goals of developing a clinical pathway and decision support tools based on clinical need and available evidence, and a protocol for linking the ED visit with community services and supports.

Work Group Process

Once oriented to the project mandate, the work group identified key issues related to children and youth with MH/A conditions. Member experts from both hospital and community settings validated the nature of concerns with access and integration of care across these settings and the importance of addressing this through a standardized care pathway. We identified the most relevant and urgent areas of concern through provincial data on the most common child and youth MH presentations.[4] A literature search yielded a paucity of relevant work in this domain. A very limited number of MH/A condition-specific clinical pathways were identified; however, these pathways were focused on chronic management of adult disorders.

Although clinical pathways typically address the assessment and management of a specific condition, the group recognized that the ED focus is primarily on risk assessment, management of crisis behaviors and disposition decisions for MH/A presentations. Consequently, we set out to develop a clinical pathway that would address these areas of focus.

Box 1
Emergency department mental health clinical pathway: Development steps

- Assemble work group.
- Identify needs and key issues.
- Literature search for existing mental health pathways.
- Environmental scan.
- Identify areas requiring improvement.
- Identify mental health/addictions screening tools.
- Determine minimum standards of care.

Environmental Scan

To gain a comprehensive understanding of how children and youth with MH/A conditions move within the ED and community MH/A services, we undertook an environmental scan of 10 EDs and 11 CMHAs across the province of Ontario. Findings from this environmental scan were notable and helped further inform our clinical pathway development with identification of several system improvements (**Table 1**).

Issue	Findings	Recommended System Improvements
Access within the ED to a child and youth crisis specialist	• Six of 10 EDs had access to pediatric crisis teams • Three of 10 EDs had access to adult crisis services for youth aged >16 y • Crisis teams were the main access link to CMHA services • Hospitals without access to a child and youth crisis clinician can transfer patient if urgent, or contact CMHA service directly	• Presence of a community worker in the ED is required to facilitate transitions
Screening tools	• Used in 2 of 10 EDs to assess children and youth with MH/A presentations • Seven of 8 remaining EDs were positive (4) or neutral (3) to their use	• Use of screening tools (self-report from youth and care-givers) and from staff assessment might improve ED staff comfort in treating this population and improve communication among EDs and CMHAs
MOA between ED and CMHAs	• Four of 10 EDs had an MOA with corresponding CMHAs; only 2 of these were aware of their existence	• Clear, up-to-date protocols required between EDs and CMHAs
Standardized crisis assessment report	• Only 1 of 10 EDs shared a standardized assessment report with corresponding CMHA • Highly variable reporting by EDs and/or CMHAs back to primary care provider	• Improved communication is required among those within the circle of care • EDs/crisis teams/CMHAs/primary care providers
Other		• EDs should have a greater role in the broader health care system • A process for patients to bypass the ED is needed

Table 1
Environmental scan of emergency departments and community mental health agencies

Abbreviations: CMHA, community mental health agency; ED, emergency department; MH/A, mental health/addictions; MOA, memorandum of agreement.

Screening Tools for Mental Health/Addictions

To guide the assessment of children and youth with MH/A presentations, the work group undertook a comprehensive search of potentially relevant screening tools for use within the ED MH clinical pathway. Through an extensive process involving input from work group members, review of a relevant report,[32] and a literature review done by Evidence In-Sight, Ontario Centre of Excellence for Child and Youth Mental Health at the Children's Hospital of Eastern Ontario,[33] 100 potential screening tools were identified addressing various MH/A conditions. We reviewed the tools for relevance, feasibility, and validity in the ED setting, because the purpose of the screening tools were for efficacy in supporting decision making for acute MH/A conditions. Based on measures of sensitivity, specificity, consistency, and reliability, 5 screening tools were selected for use within the pathway (**Table 2**). A recent systematic review was conducted since the initial selection of screening tools, and identified 3 measures as evidence-based screening options for ED physicians, two of which had already been selected for the pathway (the HEADS-ED and the Ask Suicide-Screening Questions [ASQ]).[34] This selected set of tools provide complementary information that is used to inform the physician assessment and facilitate the subsequent CMHA follow-up.

Table 2
Description of screening tools included in the EDMHCP

Screening Tool	Target Age		Description	Estimated Time for Completion	Completed/ Administered by
	<12 y	≥12 y			
Ask Suicide-Screening Questions (ASQ-5)[35,36]	—	✔	A rapid 5-item screening tool to screen youth for risk of suicide	<2 min	ED nurse
Caregiver Perception Survey (CPS)[37]	✔	—	General MH/A screening tool that addresses: • Main reason for ED visit	5–10 min	Caregiver
Youth Perception Survey (YPS)[37]	—	✔	• Other concerns • Stressors • Caregiver's perception of child's strengths/youth's perception of own strengths • Expectations for the ED visit		Youth
Pediatric Symptom Checklist (PSC-17)[38,39]	✔	—	A 17-item screening tool to facilitate recognition of cognitive, emotional and/or behavioral problems.	5–10 min	Caregiver
Global Appraisal of Individual Needs – Short Screener (GAIN-SS)[40]	—	✔	MH/A screening tool targeted for adolescents. It identifies internalizing disorders, externalizing disorders, substance use, and crime/violence	5–10 min	Youth
HEADS-ED[41,42]	✔	✔	A 7-item tool to guide ED clinician's psychosocial history to aid assessment and decision making (for ages ≥6 years)	Context dependent	ED physician MH clinician

Abbreviations: ED, emergency department; EDMHCP, emergency department mental health clinical pathway; MH/A, mental health/addictions.

Minimum Standards

As shown in **Table 3**, the work group identified a set of minimum standards of care for success.

Table 3
Emergency department mental health clinical pathway minimum standards

	Description and Rationale
Standard of Care	
1. An MOA between EDs and CMHAs	• An MOA is essential for integrated care across settings. • To ensure comprehensive understanding and organizational responsibilities within this collaboration. • The MOA template includes: ○ A statement of purpose, governing principles, details regarding the parties and processes, information sharing and privacy details.
2. 24/7 access to a child/youth MHC	• Crisis services are a main link to appropriate and timely referral to community MH services. • The child and youth MHC should contribute to the assessment, management and disposition of medium to high-risk patients, assisting with crisis deescalation and linking with CMHAs. • The child and youth MHC could be via in-person/on-site consultation, community/mobile service, telephone, or video access.
3. Standardized screening tools	• Use of screening tools inform and guide risk-based assessment in the ED. • Information shared with CMHAs can enhance communication regarding patient needs identified in the ED visit.
Practice recommendations	
4. PPO sets	• Use of standardized protocols and medications promote safe and best evidence care of patients

Abbreviations: CMHA, community mental health agency; ED, emergency department; MH, mental health; MHC, mental health clinician; MOA, memorandum of agreement; PPO, preprinted order.

THE EMERGENCY DEPARTMENT MENTAL HEALTH CLINICAL PATHWAY

The EDMH clinical pathway (EDMHCP) includes the following components:

i. An algorithm that delineates process of care within the ED from triage presentation to disposition;
ii. A set of 5 screening tools to inform the ED visit;
iii. A preprinted order set; and
iv. A documentation tool.

Each component is described further below.

Emergency Department Algorithm

As shown in **Fig. 1**, the pathway algorithm follows the typical flow of children/youth presenting to an ED with MH/A concerns. Beginning at the ED triage, patients requiring resuscitation will be immediately treated and, once stabilized, may then reenter the pathway for MH assessment. The remaining majority of patients/families will be seen by priority and asked to complete the appropriate age-based screening tools while waiting. Depending on ED resources, the patient will be assessed by a crisis worker (MH clinician) or an ED physician. The MH clinician must have an MSW, BSW, Psychological Associate, or RN degree, a knowledge of child and youth psychiatric disorders, and a minimum of 3 years of counseling experience.

ED clinicians, physicians, and nurses receive at least 2 training sessions on the screening tools and scoring. Screening tools are used to flag areas of clinical concern and a summary of the problematic areas will be used to inform the clinical assessment using the HEADS-ED. A score on the HEADS-ED tool can suggest recommendation for a MH consultation, with either psychiatry or a specialized MH clinician. After this assessment, 1 of 3 dispositions based on patient acuity and clinical judgment will be likely:

1. Immediate referral to psychiatry with potential for admission,
2. Outpatient referral for MH assessment, or
3. Follow-up with primary care provider.

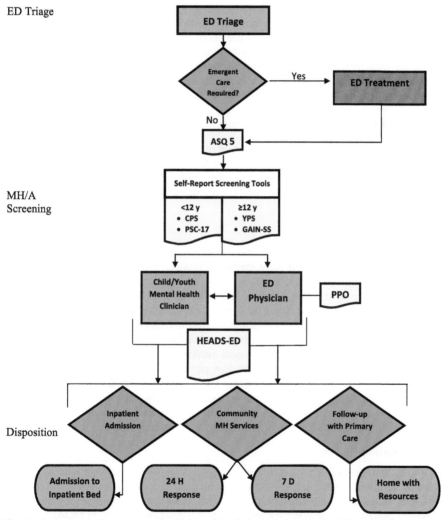

Fig. 1. Emergency department mental health clinical pathway algorithm. ED, emergency department; MH/A, mental health/addictions; Screening tools: ASQ 5, ask suicide-screening questions; C/YPS, caregiver perception survey/youth perception survey; GAIN-SS, global appraisal of individual needs-short screener; HEADS-ED, clinician screening tool; PPO, pre-printed order set; PSC-17: pediatric symptom checklist-17. (*Modified from* Jabbour M, Reid S, Polihronis C, et al. Improving mental health care transitions for children and youth: a protocol to implement and evaluate an emergency department clinical pathway. Implement Sci 2016;11(1):3; with permission.)

Preprinted Order Set

For patients requiring restraint or medications to manage agitation in the ED, a pre-printed order set is available. This order set would apply to a small percentage of patients and should only be used after deescalating strategies have been attempted.

Documentation Tool

A 1-page documentation tool for the clinical pathway is available to summarize key elements of the ED visit, including a summary of the administered screening tools and their high-risk findings, as well as disposition decisions and recommended follow-up time to establish first contact/receipt of the ED referral for CMHAs. The documentation tool is part of the patient record and gets forwarded to the relevant referring CMHA and to the primary care physician. The purpose of the tool is to facilitate communication between settings and to foster a shared approach to care provided within and between each hospital ED and CMHA partnership.

VALIDATION AND PILOT IMPLEMENTATIONS

Although our work group was representative of the relevant professionals and settings involved in care of children/youth with acute MH conditions, external validation with key stakeholder groups was essential for the pathway's acceptability and function. Modifications were made based on feedback from a series of in-person and webinar presentations with these groups.

Communities of Practice

We created virtual communities of practice to support organizations contemplating or in the early stages of pathway implementation. These webinar-based events provided the opportunity to collectively discuss implementation of the EDMHCP, address challenges, and share strategies for successful practice change. The sessions included brief presentations on experiences and reflections from implementing sites, followed by an informal question and answer period moderated by the project cochairs. These webinars attracted a large number of participants from a range of hospital- and community-based settings. Despite minimal direction and support, there was great uptake with the pathway; speaking to system needs. The pathway was intentionally flexible for adaptation to fit local needs and resource availability. We observed varied use of the screening tools, ED availability of MH clinicians, and, in some cases, persistent silos between the EDs and CMHAs. Reflections and lessons learned are provided in **Box 2**.

Implementation Toolkit

An implementation toolkit, containing a pathway overview, memorandum of agreement (MOA), and customizable tools were also developed to facilitate the recommended steps for pathway adoption.[43] An essential component to pathway adoption before beginning implementation is the development of an MOA. The purpose of the MOA is to develop a mutual understanding and outline of the specific roles and responsibilities between the hospital and CMHAs. MOAs include a brief description of the services that each CMHA provides, an overview of the process to be followed, including screening tools that the CMHA will receive from the ED, various referral procedures based on patient acuity and disposition, and follow-up response times by CMHAs (ranging from 24 hours to 7 days) to facilitate the transition from ED to community services. The complete toolkit can be found

---

Box 2
Reflections and lessons learned through communities of practice

Communities of Practice

i. Reflections
  - Community of practice webinars were important to elicit various perspectives and receive feedback on emergency department mental health clinical pathway implementation.
  - There was great uptake, despite minimal direction and support.
  - A flexible pathway was seen as important, so it could be adapted to fit local needs and resource availability.
  - There was varied use of screening tools,
  - Silos persisted between hospital EDs and CMHAs.
  - Governmental child and youth MH services restructuring had an impact on implementation.
  - Providing more MH clinician support to EDs was identified as important.
  - For successful implementation, the pathway will need to be tailored to and vary across organizations.

ii. Lessons learned and future thoughts
  - The community of practice model is helpful in exploring barriers and facilitators for implementation.
  - There are going to be variable levels of readiness for implementation across ED sites.
  - The role of technology could assist with providing support for MH distance needs (eg, telepsychiatry).
  - Alternatives to the ED need to be explored (eg, urgent care clinics).

Abbreviations: CMHA, community mental health agency; ED, emergency department; MH, mental health.

---

at http://www.pcmch.on.ca/health-care-providers/paediatric-care/pcmch-strategies-and-initiatives/ed-clinical-pathways/.

Pilot Implementations and Status

A series of pilot implementations were conducted in 5 regions throughout Ontario, and a report of the Toronto implementation has been released.[44] These pilot experiences were very helpful in both validating the need for this pathway and identifying specific activities required to tailor the pathway within each hospital–community context. The need for an integrated approach to care provided within and between each setting resonated in every pilot group. Although each pilot made different adaptations to implement the EDMHCP in their context, reports of beneficial experiences resounded from all groups. The pathway served as a vehicle to bring together and improve communication and collaboration between these typically disparate groups within each community. Sustainability seems to be related to the volume of referrals and insufficient community resources, as well as the need for ongoing support from upper level stakeholders. To further build on this experience and rigorously assess and evaluate the pathway implementation process and outcomes in different settings, we are currently conducting a mixed methods health services research project within 4 exemplar hospital–CMHA dyads.[45] Findings from this study will be reported elsewhere to further support future implementation initiatives.

SUMMARY

Throughout the process of development, dissemination, and early implementation of the EDMHCP, we have many notable observations. The most striking was in bringing together the expert work group members together and recognizing the different professional and instrumental perspectives, nomenclature/jargon and approaches to care. The development and subsequent implementation of this pathway became more of a metaphor for bringing together groups that were disconnected, and a focus for shared planning around the care of children and youth with MH/A conditions. Second, although we set out to create a clinical pathway, what we have developed is more of a service pathway, paving the paths to link services between the ED and CMHA, facilitating communication, and integrating care. Because this pathway has been received so positively, it validates the urgent need for improved service delivery for this growing population of vulnerable patients.

Our communities of practice approach was productive, with many similar conditions and challenges across communities, and hence opportunities for sharing best practices. Nevertheless, each community is unique in terms of resources, needs, and approaches. Flexibility for local adaptation is critical for successful pathway adoption.

Finally, we note that this pathway is currently focused on the ED aspect of care for children and youth presenting with acute MH conditions. Although the ED is not the ideal setting for MH/A patients, it continues to be a common entry point to MH care. Maintaining up-to-date information regarding community MH/A services is key to ensuring that the 2 systems are working in partnership. Hospital and community-based MH/A services have had difficulty keeping up with demand in the face of increasing need. Efforts to meet this need include the increasing presence of MH walk-in clinics and models of clinical service that prioritize patient need while promoting efficient patient flow (eg, Choice And Partnership Approach).[46,47] Future goals will be to evaluate the use of MH services, particularly interagency flow, for the purpose of ongoing development of CPs in child and youth MH/A care.

REFERENCES

1. Mental Health and Addictions Scorecard and Evaluation Framework (MHASEF) Research Team. The mental health of children and youth in Ontario: 2017 Scorecard. Toronto (ON): Institute for Clinical Evaluative Sciences; 2017. Available at: https://www.ices.on.ca/Publications/Atlases-and-Reports/2017/MHASEF. Accessed March 20, 2018.

2. Simon AE, Schoendorf KC. Emergency department visits for mental health conditions among US children, 2001-2011. Clin Pediatr 2014;53(14):1359–66.

3. Pittsenbarger ZE, Mannix R. Trends in pediatric visits to the emergency department for psychiatric illnesses. Acad Emerg Med 2014;21(1):25–30.

4. Canadian Institute for Health Information. Care for children and youth with mental disorders. 2015. Available at: https://secure.cihi.ca/free_products/CIHI%20CYMH%20Final%20for%20pubs_EN_web.pdf. Accessed September 28, 2017.

5. Mapelli E, Black T, Doan Q. Trends in pediatric emergency department utilization for mental health-related visits. J Pediatr 2015;167:905–10.

6. Gill PJ, Saunders N, Gandhi S, et al. Emergency department as a first contact for mental health problems in children and youth. J Am Acad Child Adolesc Psychiatry 2017;56(6):475–82.

7. Gandhi S, Chiu M, Lam K, et al. Mental health service use among children and youth in Ontario: population-based trends over time. Can J Psychiatry 2016;61:119–24.

8. Leon SL, Cloutier P, Polihronis C, et al. Child and adolescent mental health repeat visits to the emergency department: a systematic review. Hosp Pediatr 2017;7(3):177–86.

9. Larkin GL, Claassen CA, Emond JA, et al. Trends in U.S. emergency department visits for mental health conditions, 1992 to 2001. Psychiatr Serv 2005;56(6): 671–7.
10. Case SD, Case BG, Olfson M, et al. Length of stay of pediatric mental health emergency department visits in the United States. J Am Acad Child Adolesc Psychiatry 2011;50(11):1110–9.
11. Newton AS, Rathee S, Grewal S, et al. Children's mental health visits to the emergency department: factors affecting wait times and length of stay. Emerg Med Int 2014;2014:897–904.
12. Sheridan DC, Spiro DM, Fu R, et al. Mental health utilization in a pediatric emergency department. Pediatr Emerg Care 2015;31(8):555–9.
13. Dolan MA, Fein JA, The Committee on Pediatric Emergency Medicine. Pediatric and adolescent mental health emergencies in the emergency medical services system. Pediatrics 2011;127(5):e1356–66.
14. Habis A, Tall L, Smith J, et al. Pediatric emergency medicine physicians' current practices and beliefs regarding mental health screening. Pediatr Emerg Care 2007;23:387–93.
15. Ontario Ministry of Health and Long-Term Care. Open minds, healthy minds: Ontario's comprehensive mental health and addictions strategy. Ministry of Health and Long-Term Care. 2011. Available at: http://www.health.gov.on.ca/en/common/ministry/publications/reports/mental_health2011/mentalhealth_rep2011.pdf. Accessed December 14, 2017.
16. Legislative Assembly of Ontario. Select committee on mental health and addictions, interim report. Toronto: Queen's Park; 2010. Available at: http://www.ontla.on.ca/committee-proceedings/committee-reports/files_pdf/SCMHA-InterimReport-March2010.pdf. Accessed December 14, 2017.
17. Russ S, Garro N, Halfon N. Meeting children's basic health needs: from patchwork to tapestry. Child Youth Serv Rev 2010;32(9):1149–64.
18. Kinsman L, Rotter T, James E, et al. What is a clinical pathway? Development of a definition to inform the debate. BMC Med 2010;8:31.
19. Kurtin P, Stucky E. Standardize to excellence: improving the quality and safety of care with clinical pathways. Pediatr Clin North Am 2009;56(4):893–904.
20. Vanhaecht K, De Witte K, Panella M, et al. Do pathways lead to better organized care processes? J Eval Clin Pract 2009;15:782–8.
21. De Bleser L, Depreitere R, De Waele K, et al. Defining pathways. J Nurs Manag 2006;14(7):553–63.
22. Browne GJ, Giles H, McCaskill ME, et al. The benefits of using clinical pathways for managing acute paediatric illness in an emergency department. J Qual Clin Pract 2001;21:50–5.
23. Thomson P, Angus NJ, Scott J. Building a framework for getting evidence into critical care education and practice. Intensive Crit Care Nurs 2000;16(3): 164–74.
24. American Academy of Pediatrics, Committee on Pediatric Emergency Medicine, American College of Emergency Physicians, Pediatric Committee, Emergency Nurses Association Pediatric Committee. Joint policy statement—guidelines for care of children in the emergency department. Pediatrics 2009;124:1233–43.
25. Kozer E, Scolnik D, MacPherson A, et al. Using a preprinted order sheet to reduce prescription errors in a pediatric emergency department: a randomized, controlled trial. Pediatrics 2005;116:1299–302.
26. McCue JD, Beck A, Smothers K. Quality toolbox: clinical pathways can improve core measure scores. J Healthc Qual 2009;31(1):43–50.

27. Kent P, Chalmers Y. A decade on: has the use of integrated care pathways made a difference in Lanarkshire? J Nurs Manag 2006;14(7):508–20.

28. Vanhaecht K, Bollmann M, Bower K, et al. Prevalence and use of clinical pathways in 23 countries - an international survey by the European pathway association E-P-A.org. J Intgr Care Pathways 2006;10(1):28–34.

29. Darzi A. High quality care for all: NHS next stage review final report; 2008. Available at: https://www.gov.uk/government/uploads/system/uploads/attachment_data/file/228836/7432.pdf. Accessed December 14, 2017.

30. Lavelle J, Osterhoudt K, Callagham M, et al. ED Pathway for evaluation/treatment of children with behavioral health issues. Available at: http://www.chop.edu/clinical-pathway/behavioral-health-issues-clinical-pathway. Accessed December 14, 2017.

31. Langley D, Hartenstein M. Clinical pathway new or acute psych/behavioral assessments of minors (<18 years of Age). Peds Section Meeting February 2010. Available at: http://www.ohsu.edu/xd/health/services/doernbecher/programs-services/emergency/excellence/upload/clinical_pathway_acute_psych_behavioral.pdf. Accessed December 14, 2017.

32. Centre for Addiction and Mental Health. Screening for concurrent substance use and mental health problems in youth. 2009. Available at: https://www.porticonetwork.ca/web/knowledgex-archive/amh-specialists/screening-for-cd-in-youth. Accessed December 14, 2017.

33. Evidence in-sight, Ontario centre of excellence for child and youth mental health. Available at: http://www.excellenceforchildandyouth.ca/about-learning-organizations/get-ready/support-services/evidence-sight. Accessed December 14, 2017.

34. Newton AS, Soleimani A, Kirkland SW, et al. A systematic review of instruments to identify mental health and substance use problems among children in the emergency department. Acad Emerg Med 2017;24:552–68.

35. Horowitz LM, Bridge JA, Teach SJ, et al. Ask suicide-screening questions (ASQ): a brief instrument for the pediatric emergency department. Arch Pediatr Adolesc Med 2012;166(12):1170–6.

36. National Institute of Mental Health toolkit. Available at: https://www.nimh.nih.gov/news/science-news/ask-suicide-screening-questions-asq.shtml. Accessed December 14, 2017.

37. Cloutier P, Kennedy A, Maysenhoelder H, et al. Pediatric mental health concerns in the emergency department: caregiver and youth perceptions and expectations. Pediatr Emerg Care 2010;26(2):1–8.

38. Gardner W, Murphy M, Childs G, et al. The PSC-17: a brief pediatric symptom checklist with psychosocial problem subscales. A report from PROS and ASPN. Ambul Child Health 1999;5(3):225–36.

39. Murphy M, Bergmann P, Chiang C, et al. The PSC-17: subscale scores, reliability, and factor structure in a new national sample. Pediatrics 2016;138(3). https://doi.org/10.1542/peds.2016-0038.

40. Dennis ML, Chan YF, Funk RR. Development and validation of the GAIN Short Screen (GSS) for internalizing, externalizing and substance use disorders and crime/violence problems among adolescents and adults. Am J Addict 2006;15:80–91.

41. Cappelli M, Gray C, Zemek R, et al. The HEADS-ED: a rapid mental health screening tool for pediatric patients in the emergency department. Pediatrics 2012;130(2):e321–7.

42. Cappelli M, Zemek R, Polihronis C, et al. Evaluating the HEADS-ED: a brief, action oriented, clinically intuitive, pediatric mental health screening tool. Pediatr Emerg Care 2017. https://doi.org/10.1097/PEC.0000000000001180.
43. Provincial Council for Maternal and Child Health. Implementation toolkit: emergency department clinical pathway for children and youth with mental health conditions. Provincial Council for Maternal Child Health. Available at: http://www.pcmch.on.ca/health-care-providers/paediatric-care/pcmch-strategies-and-initiatives/ed-clinical-pathways/. Accessed December 13, 2017.
44. Barwick M, Boydell KM, Horning J, et al. Evaluation of Ontario's emergency department clinical pathway for children and youth with mental health conditions. Toronto: The Hospital for Sick Children; 2015. Available at: https://www.academia.edu/25456453/Evaluation_of_Ontario_s_Emergency_Department_Clinical_Pathway_for_Children_and_Youth_with_Mental_Health_Conditions. Accessed December 14, 2017.
45. Jabbour M, Reid S, Polihronis C, et al. Improving mental health care transitions for children and youth: a protocol to implement and evaluate an emergency department clinical pathway. Implement Sci 2016;11(1):1–9.
46. Robotham D, James K, Cyhlarova E. Managing demand and capacity within child and adolescent mental health services: an evaluation of the choice and partnership approach. Ment Health Rev 2010;15(3):22–30.
47. Naughton J, Basu S, O'Dowd F, et al. Improving quality of a rural CAMHS service using the choice and partnership approach. Australas Psychiatry 2015;23(5):561–5.

Maintaining Safety and Improving the Care of Pediatric Behavioral Health Patients in the Emergency Department

Fara R. Stricker, FNP-C, RN[a], Kate B. O'Neill, RN, MSN[b], Jonathan Merson, MD[c], Vera Feuer, MD[d],*

KEYWORDS

- Pediatric • Mental health • Behavioral health • Triage • Emergency departments
- Safety • Work place injury • Nursing

KEY POINTS

- The number of pediatric patients seeking care for behavioral health issues through emergency departments (EDs) is increasing. Increased volume can lead to lengthy wait times, increased aggression, and poor outcomes.
- Workflow modifications may be helpful to avoid overcrowding, delays in care and allow for safe management of this vulnerable patient population.
- The use of mental health triage tools allows for early identification of high-risk patients, supports a split-flow process, and improves outcomes by matching ED resources to specific patient needs.
- Early recognition of patients who are at high risk of harm to self or others and utilization of designated safe locations in the ED improves staff and patient safety.
- Close collaboration between emergency medicine and behavioral health departments, as well as expanding from a single consultant to a multidisciplinary team, allows for timely assessment, decreases length of stay and admission rates, and improves outcomes.

There are no conflicts of interest or disclosures.
[a] Division of Substance Abuse, Zucker Hillside Hospital, 75-59 263rd Street, Glen Oaks, NY 11004, USA; [b] Emergency Medicine Service Line, Northwell Health, 1981 Marcus Avenue, Suite 214, New Hyde Park, NY 11042, USA; [c] Behavioral Telehealth, Clinical Operations, Behavioral Health Service Line, Donald and Barbara Zucker School of Medicine at Hofstra/Northwell, 75-59 263rd Street, Glen Oaks, NY 11004, USA; [d] Division of Emergency Psychiatry, Donald and Barbara Zucker School of Medicine at Hofstra/Northwell, 75-59 263rd street, Glen Oaks, NY 11004, USA
* Corresponding author.
E-mail address: vfeuer@northwell.edu

Child Adolesc Psychiatric Clin N Am 27 (2018) 427–439
https://doi.org/10.1016/j.chc.2018.03.005
1056-4993/18/© 2018 Elsevier Inc. All rights reserved.

childpsych.theclinics.com

INTRODUCTION

Pediatric behavioral health (BH) care in the Unites States is in crisis. Although about 20% of children need mental health care, only about 20% receive the care they need.[1] A report released by the American Medical Association highlighted that there are approximately 8300 child and adolescent psychiatrists practicing in the United States, where the needs are estimated at 30,000. According to a Children's Hospital Association survey, the wait time for appointments for child and adolescent psychiatric care is almost 10 weeks, which far exceeds the prevailing benchmark for pediatric ambulatory care.[2] This is compounded by a dearth of inpatient psychiatric beds and community crisis services.[3] With an increasing demand for psychiatric care and a shortage of qualified providers, emergency departments (EDs) continue to function as the default location for patients to receive care. The ED is in fact the only treatment setting that guarantees that patients will receive an evaluation to determine if there is a psychiatric emergency, a guarantee ensured by the federal Emergency Medical Treatment and Labor Act.[3]

Most EDs are not equipped to deal with the exponential growth in the BH population. Studies have shown that patients presenting to the ED with mental health complaints have an increased chance of prolonged length of stay (LOS) and higher admission rates than patients with medical complaints.[4] The lack of expertise and resources, along with excessive volume, can lead to overcrowding, which compromises access to high-quality emergency services for the most acute patient populations and families.[3]

The ED is often a highly stimulating environment that can be countertherapeutic for patients and families. Comprehensive psychiatric assessments require lengthy interviews of parents and other collateral sources of information, which can be challenging in an ED environment characterized by limited private space and multiple distractions and disruptions. The use of dedicated areas within the ED to manage patients presenting with BH complaints is beneficial because such areas offer enhanced privacy, safety features, and a therapeutic milieu.[5]

Triage, rapid assessment, and split-flow models are well-established evidence-based strategies in emergency medicine for the improvement in flow and reduction in ED crowding.[6] These evidence-based principles can be applied to the management of BH patients in the ED.

The goal of triage is to sort and prioritize patients; that is, to assign them to resources and physical space based on their clinical need. Using a mental health triage scale improves the overall quality of care for BH patients.[7] The identification of patients at highest risk allows for the allocation of necessary resources in a timely manner, such as moving the patient to a safe space within the ED, assigning staff to monitor the patient for safety, reducing access to potentially dangerous objects, and obtaining psychiatric consultations in a timely manner.[8]

Rapid assessment by a medical or BH provider allows for the initiation of diagnostic investigations and pharmacologic or nonpharmacologic treatment early in the patient's ED stay, promoting safety, preventing escalation, and expediting decision-making regarding patient disposition. Because many ED and pediatric staff have minimal training and expertise regarding management of patients with BH complaints,[9] the completion of the rapid assessment by a BH expert can be essential in determining the needs of such patients.

Splitting off the flow of low-acuity patients to a specific care area can improve resource allocation, spare many patients from the potentially traumatic experience of a locked BH area, and prevent nonurgent care needs from obstructing patient flow in the main ED.[10] This can be optimally achieved by creating a hospital-based ambulatory crisis or urgent care model,[11] to which cases can be referred after medical screening and rapid assessment in the ED.

Another factor that can contribute to poor outcomes for BH patients is lack of training and negative attitudes on the part of the ED staff. It is noted that patients with intentional self-harm and substance use or abuse pose the greatest challenge for ED staff.[12] Providing BH education and training in modalities such as deescalation and aggression management has been shown to alleviate staff concerns and increase staff confidence and comfort in managing these patients. The adoption of multidisciplinary teams, including child and adolescent psychiatrists, social workers, BH nurses, and child life specialists, have been known to yield better outcomes for this population.[13,14] (See discussion of multidisciplinary teams and the utilization of child life, security, and BH nursing is described in more in Gary Lelonek and colleagues' article, "Multidisciplinary Approach to Enhancing Safety and Care for Pediatric Behavioral Health Patients in Acute Medical Settings," in this issue.)

This article describes how these principles have been adapted and incorporated into practice at Cohen Children's Medical Center (CCMC). This article discusses the available results of this model, as well as future directions and plans to further evaluate impact.

COHEN CHILDREN'S MEDICAL CENTER

CCMC of the Northwell Health System, anchored by a hospital with 202 inpatient beds at the border between Queens and Nassau counties, is the largest provider of pediatric health care in New York State, serving more than 1.8 million children per year. The CCMC ED currently receives more than 55,000 visits per year, with a significant and increasing percentage of patients presenting for acute and chronic BH concerns. The overall patient volume in the CCMC ED increased 2011 to 2017, with BH patients representing a consistent percentage (5%–7%) of overall ED visits.

To address this volume increase, beginning in late 2012, the hospital introduced a series of structural and operational enhancements and innovations, transitioning the care from a traditional consult model to a blended collaborative care model. Components of the model were introduced over the course of a 5-year period, as opportunities arose for workflow redesign, new infrastructure, resource reallocation, grant acquisition, and new investment in capital and personnel. These are summarized in **Fig. 1** and **Table 1** and specific elements are further described.

Physical Environment (Includes Behavioral Health Urgent Care)

Using the traditional consult model, patients with BH complaints were sent to 1 of 2 general pediatric rooms that had been stripped of dangerous items such as sinks, gases, and electrical outlets. After the 2 rooms had been filled, additional patients (up to 10 at a time) sat in hallway chairs. ED nursing was charged with maintaining situation awareness and behavioral control over a large number of patients and families at various stages of triage, assessment, disposition, and transport. It was not rare for an agitated adolescent patient brought in by armed police officers in handcuffs to share a small space with a frightened middle school student. ED nursing staff, vulnerable at baseline to workplace violence,[15] experienced an increase in their rate of injury, prompting a significant call to action.

In 2013, CCMC opened a new pediatric ED, complete with dedicated separate spaces for high-acuity and low-acuity BH patients. BH personnel were afforded the opportunity to contribute to the detailed design of the space. The high-acuity space

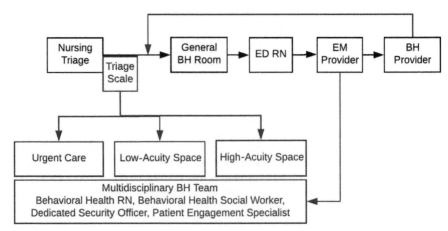

Fig. 1. Workflow transition from traditional consult model (*black*) to blended care model (*red*). EM, emergency medicine; RN, Registered Nurse.

incorporates safety recommendations and includes large rooms with barricade-proof doors, no anchoring points, secure televisions, and soothing nature-inspired artwork, an intake room for rapid assessment of newly arrived patients, a BH patient safe bathroom, a milieu area for patient overflow, a magazine-unloading station for law

Table 1
Transition to new blended care model at Cohen Children's Medical Center, by component and year of completion

Operational Components		Traditional Consult Model	New Blended Care Model	Year
Physical Environment	Acuity-specific space	None	High-acuity or low-acuity spaces	2012
	ED room design	General pediatric rooms	Pediatric BH rooms	2013
	Non-ED Space	None	BH Urgent Care Center	2017
Staff	Day or evening psychiatry staff	Mainly residents and fellows	ED-based pediatric psychiatry attendings	2013
	Social worker	General pediatric social worker	BH social worker	2013
	Security	1 officer patrolling whole ED	Dedicated officer for BH	2013
	Nursing assistant	General patient care associates	Patient engagement specialists	2015
	BH training	For select ED staff	For all ED staff	2015
	Nursing	Mainly general pediatric ED nursing	Dedicated BH nursing	2015
	Overnight psychiatry staff	Mainly residents and fellows	Attendings via telepsychiatry	2016
Triage and Flow	Provider-level rapid assessment	Emergency medicine (EM) provider toward end of ED stay	BH attending quick-look on arrival	2012
	Nursing triage scale	Medical emergency severity index 1–5	BH level 1–5 with EHR decision support	2016

enforcement, and clear lines-of-sight throughout.[5] The low-acuity space consists of a staff-monitored single-egress waiting room where several families can wait in a space that minimizes the risk for elopement without the obtrusive safety features of the high-acuity space and 2 low-acuity interview rooms for private interviews of patients and family.

In 2017, CCMC opened the BH Urgent Care Center funded by the New York State DSRIP (Delivery System Reform Incentive Payment Program) initiative, allowing for the movement of select patients out of the ED (after triage and medical screening) to this ambulatory setting for their BH evaluation. The BH Urgent Care Center is staffed by a pediatric attending psychiatrist and a licensed mental health counselor from 10:00 to 16:00 on school days, with continuous access to the ED BH provider staff. This has allowed patients and families to avoid the BH space of the ED alto-gether, a wonderful option for the many people that use the ED in nonemergencies simply for lack of access to a timely BH assessment. About one-third of patients seen in BH Urgent Care Center arrive through the ED, with the remainder walking in directly to the ambulatory program.

Staff

In the traditional consult model, most of the BH evaluations were carried out by psy-chiatry residents and fellows who received telephone supervision from pediatric psy-chiatry attending. The patients remained in the care of nurses, nursing assistants, and social workers from the pool of general pediatric staff, with a lone ED security officer checking in during patrols. BH training remained optional and was largely foregone by most staff. For ED nurses, this meant working with challenging, often volatile, BH pa-tients as part of a regular ED shift, which was itself replete with large numbers of com-plex medical patients. For nursing assistants, this meant working in very close proximity (eg, blood draws, arms-length 1-to-1 observation, crowded hallways) to potentially behaviorally unstable patients, regardless of their level of fitness and pre-paredness. Security officers, present during patrols, were frequently summoned via codes, triggered by urgent situations such as an active or impending assault on a staff member or patient.

In 2012, fellowship-trained pediatric psychiatry attendings (and their teams of nurse practitioners, fellows, or residents) began basing themselves in the CCMC ED, initially until 17:00, then 23:00, and ultimately 2:30 based on evolving analysis of volume or throughput. All attendings completed newly introduced comprehensive documenta-tion in Allscripts Sunrise Emergency Care (Raleigh, NC), providing a new departmental revenue stream and reducing the rate of inpatient insurance denials. This comprehen-sive, structured feature also allowed for quality improvement by hard-wiring care stan-dards and allowing for improved data collection. The consistent presence of pediatric psychiatry attendings permitted CCMC to serve as a telepsychiatry hub to a dozen Northwell Health System EDs between 2013 and 2016. In late 2016, Northwell opened a 24-7 telepsychiatry service out of a multispecialty telehealth center and began to cover the CCMC ED between 2:30 to 8:30.

Nonphysician BH staffing was driven by the move to the new ED and the recognition that staffing 2 larger BH areas with an ever-increasing volume, and a need to maintain safety and throughput, would require investment. On the nursing side, the proportion of the time staffed by BH nursing increased steadily, reaching 24-7 BH nursing and a midshift BH assistant nurse manager. Nursing assistants transitioned to specialized patient engagement specialists, notable for their preemployment agility testing and their extensive training in verbal and physical deescalation techniques.[16] BH social worker coverage expanded to cover 16 hours on school days. A dedicated nonroving security post was established in the high-acuity area, and all officers, as well as other staff interacting with ED BH patients, received crisis prevention training.

Triage and Flow

In the traditional consult model, BH patients were treated uniformly, regardless of their symptom severity. All BH patients received an emergency severity index level 2, whether their symptom was mild anxiety or active suicidal ideation with plan. The level of safety precautions they received (eg, wanding, searching, gowning, securing of property, placement on 1-to-1 observation) was determined by ED resources and guidelines, which were in turn subject to the variables of staffing levels and incident-driven patient safety concerns. Although some patients received safety measures commensurate with their illness severity, some high-acuity patients went undersecured, whereas many low-acuity patients felt alienated by what they experienced as disproportionately excessive interventions. Generally, the hospital erred on the side of maximal safety measures.

The Australian Triage Scale for mental health, an internationally validated nursing triage scale tying level of BH symptom severity to operational management,[17] was selected for implementation in 2015. A multistakeholder workgroup (ED, BH, information technology) convened to translate the scale into discrete radio button questions for its subsequent incorporation into the electronic health record (EHR) for real-time generation of the BH triage level. The Triage Scale enabled up-front allocation of resources to ensure safety and reduce morbidity, while minimizing the unnecessary use of high-cost resources for low-acuity patients. It also provided a mechanism to split the flow of patients from the triage location into high-acuity, low-acuity, and urgent care spaces. All of the ED nursing staff received extensive training on the scale and its underlying BH-specific knowledge base. See **Fig. 2** for details of the adopted scale and nursing actions.

The nursing triage scale is complemented by the BH attending rapid assessment or quick look. This occurs as soon as possible after the patient's arrival to the ED, and it enables not only the assignment of an acuity level but also the initiation of BH attending-level management guided by likely disposition; for example, laboratory draws and inpatient bed procurement for likely admissions.

Medical clearance is not a prerequisite to assessment by the BH team. Emergency medicine providers are assigned to the patients following triage but they perform their focused medical assessment at any point during the patient's stay. When concerns regarding comorbidities or medical stability arise, a huddle between the emergency medicine and BH providers is called to determine the needs of the patient and the ED location where the needs can best be met.

RESULTS
Impact

The changes previously described occurred over a span of 5 years and much of the data before 2012 were not available. The anecdotal and expected impact is described in **Table 2** (see later discussion of select outcome measures).

Staff Injury

Workplace violence is defined by the Office of Occupational Safety and Health Administration as violence or threat of violence (including verbal abuse and physical assaults).[18] The rate of staff injury decreased rapidly after initial interventions were implemented. The data presented here account for physical injuries but do not

BH Acuity	Patient behavioral criteria	Nursing Actions
Not triaged **Walk in**	• Identified by greeter nurse as having BH complaint or needing psychiatric evaluation • Not able to go directly from greeter RN to the RN completing the BH triage	• Continuous visual supervision until triage, do not leave patient unattended in waiting room • Metal detection or separate from belongings
Not triaged **Ambulance Bay**	• Identified by greeter nurse as having BH complaint or needing psychiatric evaluation • Not able to go directly from greeter Registered Nurse (RN) to the RN completing the BH triage	• Continuous visual supervision until triage, do not leave patient unattended, do not release EM staff until BH triage • Metal detection or separate from belongings
Un-BH triaged **Main ER**	• Patient being treated for acute medical issue that requires BH consult	• Continuous visual supervision until BH triage level is known, call BH nurse or MD to inform, proceed based on level • Metal detection/separate from belongings
Level 1 Immediate **Definite danger to life**	**Observed** • Extreme agitation or violence • Recent or observable bizarre behavior • Self destruction in the ED • Possession of a weapon • Disorientation (medical causes?) **Reported** • Verbal commands to harm self/others, patient can not resist	• Immediate CO to 1 to 1 flowsheet initiated and documented by RN • Physician (EM or BH) notification or evaluation • Code Gray (As needed) • Notify security (As needed) • If RESTRAINTS, follow P&P • Metal detection or separate from belongings • Remove clothing or search (gender sensitive, private, full skin visualized)
Level 2 - Emergency **(within 10 min)** **Probable risk of danger to self or others**	**Observed** • Patient arrives physically restrained • Extreme confusion, agitation or restlessness • Hallucinations, delusions or paranoia (patient actively experiencing symptoms) • High risk of elopement • Unable to cooperate **Reported** • Suicide attempt or serious self-harm • Threat of harm to others	• Immediate CO to 1 to 1 flowsheet initiated and documented by RN • Physician (EM or BH) notification or evaluation • Code Gray (As needed) • Notify security (As needed) • Use de-escalation techniques • Consider direct transfer to BH area after triage (NOTIFY BH) • Metal detection or separate from belongings • Remove clothing or search (gender sensitive, private, full skin visualized)
Level 3 - Urgent **(within 30 min)** **Possible danger to self or others**	**Observed** • Agitated or withdrawn • Intrusive behavior • Ambivalence about treatment **Reported** • Situational crisis • Elevated or irritable mood • Suicidal ideation or superficial self-harm • Hallucinations or delusions or paranoia	• Immediate CO to 1 to 1 flowsheet initiated and documented by RN • Physician (EM or BH) notification or evaluation • Consider direct transfer to BH area after triage (NOTIFY BH) • Metal detection or separate from belongings • Remove clothing or search (gender sensitive, private, full skin visualized)
Level 4 - Semi-Urgent **(within 60 min)** **No immediate risk to self or others**	**Observed** • Cooperative, Can articulate and assist with past history • No apparent agitation or restlessness **Reported** • Pre-existing mental health disorder • Symptoms of anxiety or depression without Suicidal ideation	• Enhanced supervision • Metal detection or separate from belongings • May stay in low-acuity area
Level 5 - NonUrgent **(within 120 min)** **No danger to self or others**	**Observed** • No acute distress, clinically well cooperative patient • No behavioral outbursts or disturbance **Reported** • Social crisis • Request for medication refill or adjustment or appointment	• Enhanced supervision • Metal detection or separate from belongings • May stay in low-acuity area

Fig. 2. Adapted Australian Triage Scale for mental health and nursing actions. CO, constant observation; P&P, policy and procedure. (*Modified from* Broadbent M, Moxham L, Dwyer T. The development and use of mental health triage scales in Australia. Int J Ment Health Nurs 2007;16(6):414; with permission.)

Table 2
Transition to new blended care model at Cohen Children's Medical Center, by impact category

Operational Components		New Blended Care Model	Impact					
			Staff Injury	Patient Injury	LOS	IM and Restraint Use	Use of 1-to-1 Observation	Patient Experience
Physical Environment	Acuity-specific space	High-acuity or low-acuity spaces	×	×	×	×	×	×
	ED room design	Pediatric BH rooms	×	×	—	—	—	×
	Non-ED space	BH Urgent Care Center	—	—	×	—	—	×
Staff	Day or evening psychiatry staff	ED-based pediatric psychiatry attendings	×	×	×	×	—	×
	Social worker	BH social worker	—	—	×	—	—	×
	Security	Dedicated officer for BH	×	×	—	×	×	×
	Nursing assistant	Patient engagement specialists	×	×	—	×	×	×
	BH training	For all ED staff	×	×	—	×	×	×
	Nursing	Dedicated BH nursing	×	×	×	×	×	×
	Overnight psychiatry staff	Attendings via telepsychiatry	—	—	×	—	×	×
Triage and Flow	Provider-level rapid assessment	BH attending quick-look on arrival	×	×	×	×	×	×
	Nursing Triage Scale	BH level 1–5 with EHR decision-support	×	×	×	×	×	×

Abbreviation: IM, intramuscular medication.

account for workplace violence through threats and verbal abuse (these rates are unavailable). The rate of ED nurse injuries is measured in relation to total number of ED visits through the following calculation to account for volume fluctuations:

$$\frac{\text{Total \# of injuries per quarter}}{\text{Total \# pts in ED per quarter}} \times 1000 \tag{1}$$

The baseline incidence of nurse injury rate averaged 0.27% (2012). After implementation of the initiatives previously described, the nurse injury rate decreased to an average of 0.05%. This improvement represents an 82% decrease in nurse injury rate. **Fig. 3** highlights the sustained improvement over a 4-year period following initial and continued process improvements.

Security Codes

The first response to potential or actual events of workplace violence is often the activation of an emergency code to alert staff and security teams of a potentially combative or assaultive person.[19] At CCMC, so-called code grays are activated by pushing a panic alarm (or by calling the hospital operator) and are announced overhead to inform staff and summon available resources to the announced location. The difficulty with these all-hands-on-deck codes is the frequent presence of excess personnel and the lack of coordination in the response. Through the process changes previously described, the use of overhead security codes reduced by 96% between 2013 and 2016 (**Fig. 4**).

Length of Stay

Clinical quality measures described by the Institute of Medicine include safety, timeliness, effectiveness, and fairness (equity).[20] ED LOS is a key metric known to correlate highly with patient satisfaction.[21] It is used as an indirect overall measure of the efficiency of the care provided. Keeping the LOS short also means reduced crowding and efficient patient flow, which helps reduce anxiety and agitation for children and families.[22] At CCMC, the LOS for BH patients who were treated and released decreased by a significant 12.5% in the 2 years following the initial interventions of rapid assessment, a blended care model, and the separating of high-acuity and

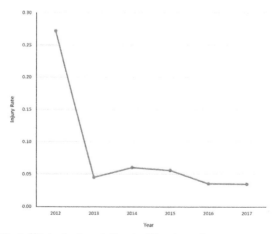

Fig. 3. Pediatric ED staff injuries in relation to ED volume by year.

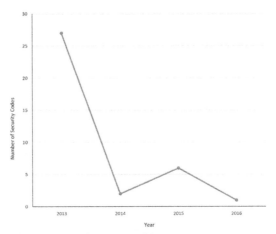

Fig. 4. Pediatric ED BH security codes activated by year.

low-acuity patients. By 2017, the LOS reduction reached 45% following interventions that included staffing changes, staff training initiatives, the introduction of the mental health nursing Triage Scale, and the opening of the BH Urgent Care Center. There was a temporary LOS increase in 2014, during a period of rapid volume growth and the construction and completion of a new ED (**Fig. 5**).

Admission Rate

The admission rate dropped by 20% (25% to 20%) between 2012 and 2014 following the introduction of the multidisciplinary team and an additional 20% (20% to 15%) in 2017 with the opening of the BH Urgent Care Center (**Figs. 6** and **7**). This reduction is aligned with national and state efforts to reduce avoidable admissions.

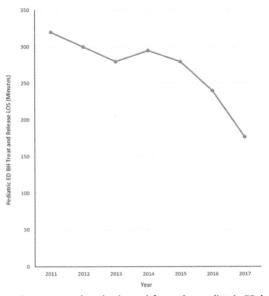

Fig. 5. LOS for BH patients treated and released from the pediatric ED by year.

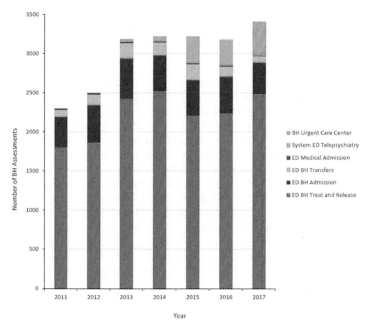

Fig. 6. Pediatric BH assessments by year and type.

Behavioral Health Urgent Care Center

Despite limited operating hours (6 hours per school day), the impact on the ED has been significant, with nearly 10% of all ED discharges triaged from the front of the ED to the BH Urgent Care Center for their assessment. Preliminary survey data

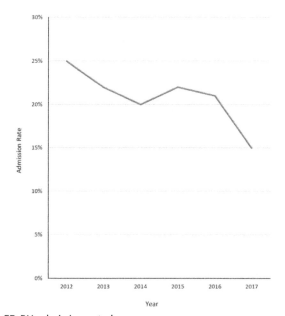

Fig. 7. Pediatric ED BH admission rate by year.

have shown a 98% rate of likeliness-to-recommend, and nearly 70% of patients reported that they would have used the ED if the BH Urgent Care Center did not exist.

SUMMARY

The current reality of inadequate inpatient, community crisis, and outpatient services for pediatric patients with BH issues in the United States positions the nation's EDs as a safety net for this vulnerable population.[23] CCMC's pediatric ED with its large catchment area spanning multiple counties in the New York metropolitan region has experienced the end-results of this crisis, yielding increasing volume and overall percentage of patients seen with BH complaints. This growth has challenged CCMC to distribute resources carefully to ensure that timely, high-quality care is not compromised and that staff members feel supported at all levels. Key components have included the use of evidence-based clinical workflows, comprehensive staff training, collaboration across disciplines, and the use of multidisciplinary teams. All improvement initiatives need to be focused, continuous, and metrics-driven to ensure change. Although CCMC had unique opportunities for investment in capital and personnel, improvement initiatives need not be costly to be successful, so long as particular attention is paid to physical layout, evidence-based workflows, and clinical team composition.

REFERENCES

1. Kataoka SH, Zhang L, Wells KB. Unmet need for mental health care among U.S. children. Am J Psychiatry 2002;159:1548–55.
2. Children's Hospital Association. Pediatric workforce shortages persist. Washington, DC: Children's Hospital Association; 2018. Available at: https://www.childrenshospitals.org/issues-and-advocacy/graduate-medical-education/fact-sheets/2018/pediatricworkforce-shortages-persist. Accessed April 11, 2018.
3. American Academy of Pediatrics. Technical report—pediatric and adolescent mental. Itasca (IL): American Academy of Pediatrics; 2011.
4. Santiago L, Tunik MG, Foltin GL, et al. Children requiring psychiatric consultation in the pediatric emergency department epidemiology, resource utilization. Pediatr Emerg Care 2006;22(2):85–9.
5. Karlin BE, Zeiss RA. Best practices: environmental and therapeutic Issues in psychiatric hospital design: toward best practices. Psychiatr Serv 2006;57(10):1376–8.
6. Jarvis PR. Improving emergency department patient flow. Clin Exp Emerg Med 2016;3(2):63–8.
7. Huckson S. Implementation of the Victorian emergency department mental health triage scale. Australas Emerg Nurs J 2008;11(2):80–4.
8. Downet L, Zun L, Burke T. Comparison of Canadian triage acuity scale to Australian emergency mental health scale triage system for psychiatric patients. Int Emerg Nurs 2015;23(2):138–43.
9. McMillan JA, Land M Jr, Leslie LK. Pediatric residency education and the behavioral and mental health crisis: a call to action. Pediatrics 2017;139(1) [pii: e20162141].
10. McGrath JL. The impact of a flexible care area on throughput measures in an academic emergency department. J Emerg Nurs 2016;41(6):503–9.
11. Gerson HA. Helping kids in crisis: managing psychiatric emergencies in children and adolescents. Arlington (VA): American Psychiatric Publishing; 2015.
12. Zun L. Care of psychiatric patients: the challenge to emergency physicians. West J Emerg Med 2016;17(2):173–6.

13. Sheridan DC, Sheridan J, Johnson KP, et al. The effect of a dedicated psychiatric team to pediatric emergency mental health care. J Emerg Med 2016;50(3): e121–8.
14. Sheridan J, Sheridan DC, Johnson KP, et al. Can't we just get some help? Providing innovative care to children in acute psychiatric crisis. Health Soc Work 2017;42(3):1.
15. Emergency Nurses Association Institute for Emergency Nursing Research. Emergency department violence surveillance study. Available at: http://www.ena.org/IENR/Documents/ENAEVSSReportAugust2010.pdf. Accessed February 24, 2011.
16. Gallo K, Smith L. Building a culture of patient safety through simulation; an interprofessional learning model [Chapter 13]. New York: Springer Publishing Company; 2014. p. 171–86.
17. Broadbent M, Moxham L, Dwyer T. The development and use of mental health triage scales in Australia. Int J Ment Health Nurs 2007;16:413–21.
18. OSHA workplace violence fact sheet. Available at: https://www.osha.gov/OshDoc/data_General_Facts/factsheet-workplace-violence.pdf. Accessed April 11, 2018.
19. Joint Commission recommendations for overhead emergency codes. Available at: https://www.jointcommission.org/assets/1/6/EM-2014_RECOMMENDATIONS_FOR_HOSPITAL_EMERGENCY_CODES_FINAL_(2).pdf. Accessed April 11, 2018.
20. Institute of Medicine. Crossing the quality chasm: a new health system for the 21st century. Washington, DC: National Academy Press; 2001.
21. Graff L. Measuring and improving quality in emergency medicine. Acad Emerg Med 2002;9(11):1091–107. Available at: www.aemj.org.
22. Sørup CM, Jacobsen P, Forberg JL. Evaluation of emergency department performance – a systematic review on recommended performance and quality-in-care measures. Scand J Trauma Resusc Emerg Med 2013;21:62.
23. Carubia B, Becker A, Levine BH. Child psychiatric emergencies: updates on trends, clinical care, and practice challenges. Curr Psychiatry Rep 2016;18:41.

Current Pediatric Emergency Department Innovative Programs to Improve the Care of Psychiatric Patients

Susan B. Roman, RN, MPH[a],*, Allison Matthews-Wilson, LCSW[a],
Patricia Dickinson, RHIT[a], Danielle Chenard, BS[b],
Steven C. Rogers, MD, MS-CTR[c]

KEYWORDS

- Care coordination • Mental health • Emergency department
- Pediatric emergency department

KEY POINTS

- For many families, emergency departments (EDs) are the first point of entry into the mental health (MH) system.
- The ED is a suboptimal environment for many children/adolescents in MH crisis.
- Establishing multidisciplinary teams within EDs to manage children with MH conditions creates opportunities for early identification, symptom recognition, and appropriate interventions, while supporting and ensuring appropriate care transitions.

The Centers for Disease Control and Prevention recognized the significance of mental health (MH) disorders among children and estimate that 22% of children have or have had a serious mental health disorder.[1–3] Although the numbers of children and adolescents with MH conditions continue to increase, only 36% receive MH services and only 40% with severe impairment receive care.[4] MH treatment of the pediatric population is often fragmented and difficult to access because of insufficient outpatient and inpatient treatment options.[5,6] Years of substandard funding has also contributed to a deficiency in qualified MH providers.[6] Barriers to accessing MH care services have resulted in inadequate provision of MH services for both adults and children in the community and often leads them to seek care in emergency departments (EDs).[7]

Disclosure Statement: No disclosures.
[a] Center for Care Coordination, Connecticut Children's Medical Center, 282 Washington Street, Hartford, CT 06106, USA; [b] Connecticut Children's Medical Center, 282 Washington Street, Hartford, CT 06106, USA; [c] University of Connecticut School of Medicine, 263 Farmington Avenue, Farmington, CT 06030, USA
* Corresponding author.
E-mail address: sroman@connecticutchildrens.org

Child Adolesc Psychiatric Clin N Am 27 (2018) 441–454
https://doi.org/10.1016/j.chc.2018.02.004
1056-4993/18/© 2018 Elsevier Inc. All rights reserved.

childpsych.theclinics.com

Approximately 6 to 9 million children are diagnosed with a significant emotional disorder, with more than half a million children presenting to the ED for treatment/stabilization of their MH condition.[8]

Child and adolescent psychiatric emergencies have been described as a national crisis.[9] The number of youth visits to EDs for MH conditions has steadily increased across the United States. Pediatric Health Information System data confirms that visits for MH conditions increased by 40% between 2009 and 2013, from an initial rate of 9.3 visits per 1000 to 13.7 visits per 1000 in 2013.[10]

As described earlier, EDs have become the safety net for a growing number of children and adolescents presenting with MH conditions. Families with children in crisis often seek treatment from EDs as their first point of entry into the MH system.[11] These patients often require care and resources beyond the capacity of most EDs.[12] In addition, EDs are highly stimulating environments that can lead to deterioration and exacerbation of symptoms, especially for patients with complicated mental illness. For most patients with MH, the ED is a suboptimal environment during times of crisis.[13]

The American Academy of Pediatrics recently published 2 clinical reports offering guidance to pediatric ED (PED) clinicians caring for children in MH crisis. The guidelines (part I and II) provide educational support in addressing common clinical challenges and emphasizes the importance of discharge planning and specifically suggests coordinating care with the medical home on discharge.[14,15] Although many clinical reports and guidelines address the issues of provider competency in caring for children with MH conditions, there is limited evidence-based practices to address the increasing numbers of children/adolescents presenting to the ED in crisis. Most of these children/adolescents are discharged from the ED, but return visits are common. Recidivism rates ($\approx$45%) can be attributed to a variety of known risk factors, including female sex, mood disturbances, use of psychotropic medications, past and present utilization of MH services, the social determinants of health, and involvement in the child welfare system.[16,17] However, less is known about the difficulty in accessing and securing follow-up MH services and its impact on ED utilization and recidivism. EDs that can facilitate early interventions and linkages to MH services and community resources may potentially reduce subsequent crisis, reduce recidivism rates, and most importantly have a profound influence on short- and long-term behavioral health outcomes.[6]

It is recommended that EDs develop feasible, site-based interventions for MH patients that will improve linkage to community services and resources. Collaboration among ED providers, public health agencies, MH providers, and other stakeholders is critical to generating a body of best practices for ED-based acute psychiatric care.[18]

Establishing multidisciplinary teams within the ED to manage children with MH conditions creates opportunities for early identification, symptom recognition, and appropriate interventions, while supporting appropriate care transitions.[19] Increasing linkages to MH services following ED discharge is crucial for children, especially those presenting with suicidality.[20,21]

In an effort to address MH access and improve quality and efficient management of children/adolescents burdened with MH conditions, the authors describe ED projects that target this vulnerable population. Five North American hospitals/health care systems volunteered to feature ED projects that address postdischarge follow-up for pediatric MH emergencies: Allina Health, Nationwide Children's Hospital, Children's Hospital of Eastern Ontario, Connecticut Children's Medical Center, and Rhode Island Hospital. The authors surveyed each site on the following: project descriptions/histories, goals, data/results, and lessons learned. The authors think that this information will help stimulate discussions and inspire innovations that will inform the design of more comprehensive ED programs that will support the diverse needs of children and their families during and after an ED visit for MH crisis.

PROJECT DESCRIPTIONS

Team: Lifespan Partners: Emma Pendleton Bradley Hospital (Bradley), Hasbro Children's Hospital (HCH), Gateway Healthcare (Gateway)
  Location: Providence, Rhode Island
  Project title: Kids'Link Hotline
  Funding: Substance Abuse and Mental Health Services Administration (SAMHSA) Cooperative Agreements for Youth Suicide Prevention (Garrett Lee Smith Memorial Act) and a grant from the Rhode Island Foundation
  Lifespan has several sites offering psychiatric emergency services (PES) for children: Bradley is a children's psychiatric hospital providing care to those with psychological, developmental, and behavioral problems, offering a wide range of treatment programs. The Bradley Access Center provides urgent evaluations for children in crisis as well as a crisis hotline called Kids'Link. HCH, the pediatric division of Rhode Island Hospital, includes an ED that receives consultative services through a specialized PES team composed of a licensed independent clinical social worker, MH clinicians, advanced practice nurses, and doctors. Gateway offers many community-based MH services for adults and children, including PES.
  In 2015, the pediatric PES teams from these 3 partners became a unified service under central leadership, with cross-training of clinicians at multiple sites. Now Lifespan Pediatric Behavioral Health Emergency Services (LPBHES), with its varied types and locations of emergency services operating as one team, provides improved coordination of these services creating optimal use of limited resources. A goal of LBPHES has been to expand utilization of Kids'Link as the front door to the service, to increase early access to care, improve families' experience with a complex MH care system within Rhode Island, and divert from the HCHED those patients who do not absolutely require management in an ED.
  Using Kids'Link as the LPBHES triage line gives clinicians the opportunity to work with callers to determine the appropriate timing and type of evaluation needed, directing them to the most appropriate site, rather than families, schools, and providers thinking that their only option is to send children to an ED. Enhanced marketing of the Kids'Link line was implemented with the goal to increase use by families, schools, and providers.
  In 2014, Bradley partnered with the Rhode Island Department of Health and Rhode Island Student Assistance Services, via a SAMHSA-funded grant to address the needs of school systems who must manage children in MH crisis with limited resources and training. This initiative has 4 components:

1. Starting in March 2015, to standardize the assessments of students at risk for harm to themselves or others, school crisis teams are trained to include a screening tool developed based on the Columbia Suicide Severity Rating Scale.
2. New crisis procedures are implemented within schools so they contact Kids'Link to review the results of this screening tool.
3. Information provided by the screening tool gives the Kids'Link clinician necessary data to inform appropriate disposition decisions. When possible, these children can be connected directly with the appropriate level of care. When a full evaluation is still required to determine appropriate services, the clinician will help the school decide where and when an urgent evaluation should occur. Whenever possible, an ED evaluation and emergency medical services transport are avoided.

4. With consent, Bradley Access staff provide follow-up contact with at-risk students at 2 weeks, 3 months, and 1 year after their crisis. Follow-up calls are intended to screen for any barriers to treatment engagement for at-risk youths and to provide alternatives if treatment has not yet started.

This initiative has recently begun to train pediatricians in the use of the suicide screening tool and encourage them to use Kids'Link for information about ideal emergency evaluation locations and resources available to support their patients.

Now starting year 4 of the 5-year SAMHSA-funded initiative, school and pediatrician trainings on screening and use of Kids' Link have shown progress. Kids'Link received less than 2500 calls during fiscal year (FY) 2015 and is now on track to receive nearly 6000 calls by the end of FY 2017. The feedback from schools and enrolled families has been universally positive. Services provided have improved communication between schools and MH professionals and improved coordination and outcomes of patient care. Although Kids'Link calls significantly increased, MH visits in the ED have remained fairly steady, though ED staff report an increase in acuity. This finding would be expected as Kids'Link calls increase, indicating LBPHES is helping a wider group of patients overall, yet increasingly only sending the most acute to the ED. An analysis of the current data from FY 2017 demonstrated that of the nearly 6000 crisis calls, only 4.65% were instructed to go to the ED.

Because of significantly increased call volume, in 2016 LPBHES applied for and received a Rhode Island Foundation Grant in order to increase efficiency and standardize the phone triage work being done through Kids'Link. This project launched in January 2017 and will include the development of a standardized, interactive triage tool to ultimately be included in the electronic health record. The project also includes chart reviews to determine, among other things, who is currently using Kids'Link and for what reasons, to provide information so that LPBHES can enhance marketing to reach those populations not currently engaging with its phone triage services.

Team: Nationwide Children's
Location: Columbus, Ohio
Project title: Outpatient Crisis Program
Funding: none

Nationwide Children's Hospital developed this innovative program approximately 10 years ago to address an increase in high-risk MH/behavioral health children and adolescents up to 18 years of age, seen in clinical settings within Nationwide Children's Hospital. In response to the increasing volume of youths needing behavioral/MH treatment and the need to have urgent response capabilities, Nationwide Children's created an Outpatient Crisis Program to support their high-risk patients with urgent assessments and acute response availability. For example, internal data from 2016 was notable for the hospital having 180,165 behavioral health visits in their outpatient clinics. The Outpatient Crisis Program works with the hospital's Behavioral Health Intake Department to triage new patients to determine who requires an urgent assessment. Urgent is described as requiring an assessment within 72 hours. The program assists other staff at Nationwide Children's through assessment, consultation, safety planning, and assistance with hospitalization when patients are experiencing a MH crisis. In addition, licensed therapists provide short-term therapy to individuals and families who are waiting to be connected to an ongoing provider (referred to as bridging therapy). The Outpatient Crisis Program will manage a child's care on discharge until appropriate level-of-care services are identified. The development of the Outpatient Crisis Program at Nationwide Children's has allowed for quick linkage for youths needing an urgent assessment to decrease ED visits and provide bridging treatment of youths stepping down from a higher level of care during high-risk times. From December 1, 2016 to November 30, 2017, the Nationwide Children's Behavioral Health Outpatient Crisis Program saw a total of 3880 completed appointments; 1778 of those were unique visits. Out of the 3880 appointments, 43% or 767 appointments (763 unique patients) were able to be diverted from the ED and seen urgently by the Outpatient Crisis Program. When patients are seen in the most appropriate level of care, it is a significant benefit to patients and families as well as the organization.

Team: Children's Hospital of Eastern Ontario (CHEO)

Location: Ontario, Canada

Project title: Crisis Management Following Emergency Department Visits using the HEADS-ED Screening Tool

Funding: Public Health Agency of Canada

CHEO began with a study funded from 2015 to 2016 by the Public Health Agency of Canada. CHEO looked at the increase of MH-afflicted pediatric patients seeking emergency treatment as a first point of entry and reentry into the health care system. They found that parents expected ED staff to assess and manage their children's MH needs[22] and then connect them to long-term community MH supports.

CHEO worked to create and validate a Home, Education, Activities and peers, Drugs and alcohol, Suicidality, Emotions and behavior and Discharge resources (HEADS-ED) rapid MH screening tool. This brief tool can easily be adopted into a normal PED workflow[23] by helping ED professionals take a psychosocial history and using the information to facilitate decisions around patient disposition and discharge.[24,25]

CHEO created a Web site (www.ottawa.heads-ed.com) in partnership with a local MH resource and assistance directory (www.ementalhealth.ca) to provide recommendations for community MH services based on the areas of need identified in the HEADS-ED evaluation. The goals of both the Web site and the HEADS-ED evaluation were to help (1) ED physicians to screen for MH-related concerns and with disposition decision-making and (2) increase patient linkage and connection with appropriately matched community MH services within 30 days of an ED visit. Secondary objectives included a decrease in length of stay (LOS) in the ED, decreased repeat visits, and increased patient satisfaction with their ED visit and discharge recommendations. Preliminary analyses on a subset of 250 patients demonstrated that clinician uptake of the Web-based HEADS-ED tool to screen for MH concerns in the ED was 84% (n = 211 of 250). There were fewer consultations to psychiatry when the HEADS-ED was used (25%; n = 52 of 211) compared with when it was not (46%; n = 18 of 39; $P = .006$). Of the patients who were discharged from the ED and reached for 1-month follow-up, 74% of caregivers and youths (n = 60 of 81) were able to obtain at least 1 recommended service when physicians completed the HEADS-ED. Further analyses are underway using the full dataset to determine if HEADS-ED screening improves patient linkage to appropriately matched community services.

Team: Allina Health System

Location: Minnesota

Project title: Washburn Allina Acute Response Model (WAARM)

Funding: Initial start-up funds from the Abbott Northwestern Hospital general fund; ongoing support from the Abbott Northwestern Hospital Foundation in Minneapolis MH fund; providers bill for MH services provided where possible

Allina Health is a Minnesota-based integrated health system, the largest provider of MH services in the state. Allina Health hypothesized that a lack of immediate access to in-home crisis stabilization services has led to an increased use of PED services, longer boarding times in the PED for children and adolescents with a MH presentation, as well as overall MH admissions to the hospital inpatient units. The goal of WAARM is to provide immediate access to in home services following the first contact with the PED. Allina Health specifically identified the Twin Cities metro area of Minneapolis and Saint Paul as the area in which the challenges were most pronounced, though they acknowledge this increase in pediatric MH issues is a statewide concern. The goal of the WAARM pilot project is to reduce MH stays and boarding in the Allina PED by increasing access and referral of children in the PED to the Washburn Center for Children. Allina created a pilot program in which MH clinicians in the PED partnered with a well-known community MH care provider of in-home crisis stabilization service, Washburn Center for Children, to allow immediate access to this service. Previous wait times for crisis services were as long as 4 weeks. Currently, patients can be seen for an immediate evaluation by a crisis worker in the ED, who will schedule an in-home session within 72 hours after discharge from the ED. If the crisis worker is not in the ED, a referral will be made and a follow-up with patients and families will occur within 24 hours.

The project goals were decreasing PED visit times and increasing appropriate discharge plans from the PED, avoiding unnecessary hospitalizations. The crisis stabilization team will offer families a short-term, 5-session crisis intervention: one warm handoff (a face-to-face contact with dedicated licensed crisis clinician on site or via telehealth) and 4 additional crisis stabilization sessions in the community. The crisis clinician, a licensed independent clinical social worker with crisis and family experience, will support Allina Health full time and be available in the ED for immediate referrals and will also meet with patients and families for scheduled sessions in the community.

Patients will also be referred for additional MH services as needed. If necessary, clients can then be referred to Washburn's' long-term crisis stabilization treatment (up to 6 months). Outcome measures for the project, which began during the writing of this article, includes length of visit in the ED, percentage of children and adolescents safely discharged home, data on return visits to the ED, and overall patient/family satisfaction.

Team: Connecticut Children's Medical Center

Location: Hartford, Connecticut

Project title: Enhanced Care Coordination (ECC) for Youth with MH Chief Complaints in a PED

Funding: Connecticut Children's Medical Center (CT Children's)–Office for Community Child Health (OCCH), Connecticut Department of Children and Families (DCF)

The Center for Care Coordination (center) at CT Children's provides care coordination (CC) and community linkage for all children and youths, 0 to 21 years of age. The center partnered with the PED's behavioral health unit to develop an ECC pilot that began in the fall of 2015. Master in social work (MSW) clinical care coordinators were connected with families whose children were evaluated and deemed safe for discharge to home. Inclusion criteria was limited to children/youth between 0 and less than 18 years of age not known to the center, residing in its catchment area, and without involvement in the child welfare system. Within 48 hours after discharge, clinical care coordinators contacted families for services. Coordination involves a comprehensive needs assessment, a review of current services/resource utilization, PED discharge recommendations support in accessing and securing critical medical and behavioral health follow up care, as well as supporting families in addressing any educational needs or modifications and social support services. The authors' primary goal was to ensure feasibility of this program, so outcome measures included efficiency (defined as total number of children cared for by PED-SW and LOS) and connectivity (defined as number of children engaged in ECC with communication of the discharge plan to community providers).

Data were entered into the Windows ACCESS 2016 database in order to help demonstrate feasibility and allow for ongoing quality-improvement measures as follows:

1. Demographic data
2. Data specific to each encounter
   o Time spent per encounter
   o Focus of the encounter
   o Type of activity (written, meeting, phone, forms processing, writing care plan, and case review)
   o Provider of services (parent/patient, primary care provider, medical specialist, community, state or private agency, behavioral clinician, school, or allied health)
   o Patient needs (assessed and categorized into the following focus of encounters: advocacy, basic needs, education, finance, interagency coordination, legal, medical/dental, behavioral/MH, social connections, and transition to adult health care)
3. Communication of care plan and linkages (phone calls, emails, faxes).

The total PED volume was 4% lower in 2015 (14,434) compared with 2014 (15,072), but 18% more patients presented to the PED with MH chief complaints in 2015. PED-SW cared for 70% more MH patients in 2015 (218, 23%) versus 2014 (128, 16%). The average LOS for PED-SW patients remained unchanged (approximately 3 hours). PED-SW identified that 32% (69 of 218) of their MH patients met the criteria (**Table 1**) and were referred to CC, but 33% (23 of 69) did not respond and 5 additional patients were excluded. To communicate the care plan, CC staff engaged (phone calls, e-mails, faxes) with community providers 339 times (**Fig. 1**). CC engaged with the educational system 2.7 episodes per child (average) and with MH providers 2.9 episodes per child (average); 100% of primary care physicians were connected and received information about the patient care plans.

The authors concluded that ECC for PED MH patients is feasible. PED social worker efficiency improved as demonstrated by increased patients seen and similar LOS compared with the same time period last year without CC. Patient/family engagement with ECC and connectivity to PCP, school, and MH providers were ensured. The program is following a continuous quality-improvement model with future activities being

Table 1 Demographics	
Quality Improvement Project Phase 1: Feasibility	
October–December 2015	ECC patients (n = 69)
Male (%)	48 (70)
Female (%)	21 (30)
Mean Age (y)	10.9
Ethnicity (%)	
White	21 (30)
African American	13 (19)
Hispanic	21 (30)
Other/unknown	14 (20)

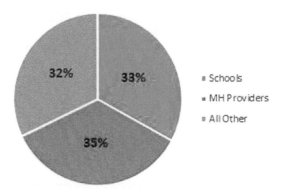

Fig. 1. Percentage of connectivity of children with community providers.

developed/conducted to determine the cost-effectiveness and relative patient bene-fits/outcomes (recidivism rates, patient/family satisfaction) when MH patients are enrolled in ECC before discharge from a PED.

Discussion

The Kids'Link program and the Outpatient Crisis Program help to identify, refer, and treat before patients even arrive in the ED. These programs promote coordination, including interagency community-based coordination, a strategic approach to increasing access for children needing services,[24,25] and helps to prevent unneces-sary ED visits. CHEO's program, Crisis Management following Emergency Depart-ment Visits using the HEADS-ED Screening Tool, helps to ensure efficient care for MH patients while in PEDs as well as by supporting connection to community MH ser-vices. Finally, Connecticut Children's ECC and the WAARM ensures connection to services following an ED visit. These 5 programs uniquely address the MH challenges presenting at their institutions; their similarities/differences are illustrated in **Tables 2** and **3**.

Children with MH conditions, like children with complex medical needs, are consid-ered a highly vulnerable population requiring cross-sector integration of service and resource providers. CC and programs such as those described here support families and patients by identifying and linking them to essential community services and re-sources.[26] Coordinating care is considered an essential component of providing care to children and youths with MH conditions.[27] Approximately 40% of families hav-ing children with an MH condition report a need for help with coordinating their child's care because 41% of their needs went unmet.[28] Adopting and/or strengthening these types of services and family centered care could result in more efficient and effective care for all children and adolescents affected by MH conditions.[29] In addition, these programs may reduce unnecessary ED visits and recidivism, which would lessen the burden on already busy PEDs.

Limitations

This article is a descriptive commentary of site-specific ED models developed to address the unprecedented number of children and adolescents being admitted to the ED in MH crisis. The authors introduction of novel programs demonstrates the need to reconsider how we provide care to this vulnerable group of patients within the ED. This review is not a comprehensive review of PED/ED-embedded programs but an opportunity to begin the conversation on how to shift the paradigm of care

Table 2
Comparison of programs (Lifespan, Nationwide, Children's Hospital of Eastern Ontario)

Hospital	LPBHES: Bradley Hospital, Hasbro Children's, Gateway Healthcare	Nationwide Children's	CHEO
Project title	Kids'Link Hotline	Outpatient Crisis Program	Crisis Management following Emergency Department Visits using the HEADS-ED Screening Tool
Identified challenge	• Several sites offering psychiatric services	• Increase in high-risk MH/behavioral health adolescents seen in clinical settings within children's hospital	• There is an increase of MH patients seeking ED treatment as first point of entry. • Parents expected the ED to assess and manage child's MH needs.
Action taken	• Become a unified service under central leadership.	• Create an outpatient crisis program to support high-risk patients with urgent assessments and acute response availability.	• Create and validate HEADS-ED rapid mental health screening tool • Created a Web site that provides recommendations based on the need identified in the HEADS-ED.
Goal	• Improve coordination of services with optimal use of limited resources. • Expand Kids'Link as the front door to services. • Increase early access to care. • Improve the family experience.	• Triage new patients to determine who requires urgent assessment (within 72 h). • Licensed therapists provide short-term therapy to those waiting to be connected to an ongoing provider. • Psychiatry and crisis stabilization team create a bridge discharge. • Ensure a connection to postdischarge behavioral health care.	• ED to screen for MH concerns and with disposition decision-making • Increase patient linkage and connection with community MH services within 30 d of ED visit • Decrease LOS • Decrease repeat visits • Increase patient satisfaction

(continued on next page)

Table 2
(continued)

Hospital	LPBHES: Bradley Hospital, Hasbro Children's, Gateway Healthcare	Nationwide Children's	CHEO
Method	• Expand utilization of Kids'Link as the front door to services. • Increase early access to care. • Improve the family experience of the complex MH care system.	• Licensed therapists provide short-term therapy for those waiting to be connected to an ongoing provider (bridging therapy). • Manage a child's care on discharge until appropriate level of care services identified.	• Help PED professionals take psychosocial history and use info to facilitate decisions about patient disposition and discharge. • Provide recommendations of community MH services based on the need identified in the HEADS-ED.
Outcome	• Standardize assessments • School crisis teams trained to include screening tool • New crisis procedures implemented within schools • Follow-up contact with at-risk students at 2 wk, 3 mo, and 1 y after crisis • Divert from HCH-ED those patients who do not absolutely require management there	• Development of the program has allowed for quick linkage for youths needing urgent assessment to decrease ED visits. • Provide bridging treatment of youths stepping down from a higher level of care during high-risk times.	
Data/results	• Improved coordination of services creating optimal use of limited resources • Improved communication between schools and MH professionals		

Table 3
Comparison of programs (Connecticut Children's/Allina health)

Hospital	Connecticut Children's	Allina Health
Project title	ECC for Youth with Mental Health Chief Complaints in a PED	Home Crisis Stabilization Team
Challenge identified	• Improve linkage to community services and resources • Collect data on its impact on ED utilization and recidivism	• Increase in child/adolescent MH visits in ED
Action taken	• ED behavioral health unit partnered with the center to develop an ECC pilot • MSW clinical care coordinators connected with children with an ED disposition to home	• Dedicated home crisis stabilization team partnered with well-known community MH provider
Goal	• Ensure feasibility of this program so outcome measures included efficiency (defined as total number of children cared for by PED-SW and LOS) and connectivity (defined as number of children engaged in ECC and communication of the discharge plan to community providers)	• Decrease ED visit times • Increase appropriate discharge plans • Avoid unnecessary hospitalizations
Method	• Within 48 h after discharge, clinical care co-ordinators contacted families for services. • Coordination involves a comprehensive needs assessment, a review of current services/resource utilization and PED discharge recommendations, and support in accessing and securing critical medical and behavioral health care and critical educational and community services.	• Offer families a short-term 5-session crisis intervention • 1 intake/evaluation and 4 additional sessions
Outcome	• The program is following a continuous quality-improvement model. • Future activities are being developed/conducted to determine the cost-effectiveness and relative patient benefits/outcomes (recidivism rates, patient/family satisfaction) when MH patients are enrolled in ECC before discharge from a PED.	• Pending
Data/results	• 100% of PCPs received care plan information. • Care coordinators connected to community providers 339 times. • Each child had an average 2.7 connections to school and 2.9 connections to MH providers.	• Evaluation goals pending: decrease visit stays in ED • % patients discharged home • Data on return ED visits • Overall patient satisfaction survey results

to effectively manage children/families. Additional research on these and other innovative MH models is critical in determining best practices.

SUMMARY

Transformation of pediatric behavioral health care requires innovation. To address the needs of children/families, as well as the myriad of challenges faced by EDs, we must continue to design and disseminate models that enable children and their families to access the right care, at the right time and at the right place. EDs can no longer function solely as an entity to provide crisis intervention; the ability to link children/families to community services and resources is critical.[30] Reallocating resources, building capacity, and developing and strengthening community partnerships that focus on care before, during, and after ED visits are essential in reducing MH-related visits. Site-based ED interventions that not only triage and stabilize children in crisis but create opportunities for enhanced support and coordination seem promising.

To further the goal of improving emergent MH care for children, these 5 North American sites have agreed to convene a learning collaborative to develop best practices and quality metrics. Discussions will focus on evidence-based practices, ongoing research, and informing health policy.

Note: To learn more and participate please see www.childrensemergencymentalhealth. org.

REFERENCES

1. The National Institute of Mental Health: Available at: https://www.nimh.nih.gov/health/statistics/prevalence/any-disorder-among-children.shtml. Accessed July 7, 2017.

2. Merikangas KR, He JP, Burstein M, et al. Lifetime prevalence of mental disorders in U.S. adolescents: results from National Comorbidity Survey Replication—Adolescent Supplement (NCS-A). J Am Acad Child Adolesc Psychiatry 2010; 49(10):980–9.

3. Pittsenbarger Z, Mannix R. Trends in pediatric visits to the emergency department for psychiatric illness. Acad Emerg Med 2014;21:25–30.

4. Chun TH, Duffy SJ, Linakis JG. Emergency department screening for adolescent mental health disorders: the who, what, when, where, why, and how it could and should be done. Clin Pediatr Emerg Med 2013;14(1):3–11.

5. Dolan MA, Fein JA, and the Committee on Pediatric Emergency Medicine. American Academy of Pediatrics, technical report-pediatric and adolescent mental health emergencies in the emergency service system. Available at: www.pediatrics.org/cgi/doi/10.1542/peds.2011-0522. Accessed July 26, 2017.

6. Newton AS, Ali S, Johnson DW, et al. Who comes back? Characteristics and predictors of return to emergency department services for pediatric mental health care. Acad Emerg Med 2010;17:177–86.

7. Centers for Disease Control and Prevention (CDC). Emergency department visits by patients with mental health disorders — North Carolina 2008–2010. MMWR Morb Mortal Wkly Rep 2013;62(23):469–72. Available at: https://www.cdc.gov/mmwr/preview/mmwrhtml/mm6223a4.htm. Accessed July 28, 2017.

8. Sheridan D, Spiro D, Fu R, et al. Mental health utilization in a pediatric emergency department. Pediatr Emerg Care 2015;31(8):555–9.

9. Rogers SC, Griffin LC, Masso PD, et al. CARES: improving the care and disposition of psychiatric patients in the pediatric emergency department. Pediatr Emerg Care 2015;31(3):173–7.

10. Rogers S, Mulvey C, Divietro S, et al. Escalating mental health care in pediatric emergency departments. Clin Pediatr (Phila) 2017;56(5):488–91.

11. Jabbour M, Reid S, Polihronis C, et al. Improving mental health care transitions for children and youth: a protocol to implement and evaluate an emergency department clinical pathway. Implement Sci 2016;11(1):90.

12. Christodulu KV, Lichenstain R, Weist MD, et al. Psychiatric emergencies in children. Pediatr Emerg Care 2002;18(4):268–70.
13. Dolan MA, Fein JA, and the Committee on Pediatric Emergency Medicine. American Academy of Pediatrics, technical report-pediatric and adolescent mental health emergencies in the emergency service system. Available at: www.pediatrics.org/cgi/doi/10.1542/peds.2011-0522. Accessed April 11, 2018.
14. Chun T, Mace S, Katz E, et al. Executive summary: evaluation and management of children and adolescents with acute mental health or behavioral problems. Part 1: common clinical challenges of patients with mental health and/or behavioral emergencies. Pediatrics 2016;10:1542–71.
15. Chun T, Mace S, Katz E, et al. Evaluation and management of children and adolescents with acute mental health or behavioral problems. Part II: recognition of clinically challenging mental health related conditions presenting with medical or uncertain symptoms. Pediatrics 2016;138(10):1542–73.
16. Leon SL, Cloutier P, Polihronis C, et al. Child and adolescent mental health repeat visits to the emergency department: a systematic review. Hosp Pediatr 2017;7(3):177–86.
17. Cloutier P, Thibedeau N, Barrowman N, et al. Predictors of repeated visits to emergency department crisis intervention program. CJEM 2017;19(2):122–30.
18. Larkin G, Beautrais A, Spirito A, et al. Mental health and emergency medicine: a research agenda. Acad Emerg Med 2009;16(11):1110–9.
19. Baren JM, Mace SE, Hendry PL, et al. Children's mental health emergencies-part 1: challenges in care: definition of the problem, barriers to care, screening, advocacy, and resources. Pediatr Emerg Care 2008;24(6):399–408.
20. Grupp-Phelan J, Delgado SV, Kelleher KJ. Failure of psychiatric referrals from the pediatric emergency department. BMC Emerg Med 2007;7:12.
21. MacWilliams K, Curran J, Racek J, et al. Barriers and facilitators to implementing the HEADS ED: a rapid screening tool for pediatric patients in emergency department. Pediatr Emerg Care 2016. https://doi.org/10.1097/PEC.0000000000000651.
22. Cappelli M, Gray C, Zemek R, et al. The HEADS-ED: a rapid mental health screening tool for pediatric patients in the emergency department. Pediatrics 2012;130(2):130.e1-7.
23. Cappelli M, Zemek R, Polihronis C, et al. Evaluating the HEADS-ED: a brief, action oriented, clinically intuitive, pediatric mental health screening tool. Pediatr Emerg Care 2017. https://doi.org/10.1097/PEC.0000000000001180.
24. Sarvet B, Gold J, Bostic JQ, et al. Improving access to mental health care for children: the Massachusetts Child Psychiatry Access Project. Pediatrics 2010;126(6):1191–200.
25. Winters NC, Pumariga A, Work Group on Community Child and Adolescent Psychiatry, Work Group on Quality Issues. Practice parameter on child and adolescent mental health care in community systems of care. J Am Acad Child Adolesc Psychiatry 2007;46(2):284–99.
26. Lipkin PH, Alexander J, Cartwright JD, et al. Care coordination in the medical home: integrating health and related systems of care for children with special health care needs. Pediatrics 2005;5:1238–44.
27. Jorina M, Cammaerts A, Singer J, et al. Advancing the measurement of care coordination in pediatric behavioral health. J Dev Behav Pediatr 2016;37:674–84.
28. Brown N, Green J, Desai M, et al. Need and unmet need for care coordination among children with mental health conditions. Pediatrics 2014;133(3):e530–7.

29. Adams SH, Newacheck PW, Park MJ, et al. Medical home for adolescents: low attainment rates for those with mental health problems and other vulnerable groups. Acad Pediatr 2013;13(2):113–21.
30. Cloutier P, Kennedy A, Maysenhoelder H, et al. Pediatric mental health concerns in the emergency department. Pediatr Emerg Care 2010;26(2):99–106.

Social Services and Behavioral Emergencies
Trauma-Informed Evaluation, Diagnosis, and Disposition

Patrick J. Heppell, PsyD[a,b,]*, Suchet Rao, MD[c,d]

KEYWORDS

- Child welfare • Child and adolescent trauma • Psychiatric emergency
- Pediatric mental health

KEY POINTS

- Children and adolescents involved in the child welfare system are more likely to have experienced abuse and neglect.
- Mental health professionals evaluating children and adolescents involved in the child welfare system should be familiar with the relevant legal and confidentiality-related issues.
- Historical information from a wide variety of sources, a child's current presentation in the emergency room (ER) and factors that led both to their involvement with the child welfare system and to their current ER visit should all be taken into consideration when making diagnostic and disposition decisions.
- A trauma-informed approach increases the likelihood of arriving at an accurate diagnosis, and thus results in more appropriate and useful pharmacologic and psychosocial treatments.

The authors do not have any relationship with a commercial company that has a direct financial interest in subject matter or materials discussed in the article.
[a] Department of Child and Adolescent Psychiatry, Hassenfeld Children's Hospital, NYU Langone, Child Study Center, One Park Avenue, 7th Floor, New York, NY 10016, USA; [b] Mental Health Team, Nicholas Scoppetta Children's Center, New York, NY, USA; [c] Department of Child and Adolescent Psychiatry, Hassenfeld Children's Hospital, NYU Langone, New York, NY, USA; [d] Psychiatry and Behavioral Health, NYC Administration for Children's Services, 150 William Street, 11th Floor, New York, NY 10038, USA
* Corresponding author. Department of Child and Adolescent Psychiatry, Hassenfeld Children's Hospital, NYU Langone, Child Study Center, One Park Avenue, 7th Floor, New York, NY 10016.
E-mail address: Patrick.heppell@nyumc.org

A caseworker accompanies a quiet girl to the psychiatric ER and reports: "Jessica is a 9-year-old girl who got herself kicked out of 3 foster homes in the past 4 months. At first, we thought she was just sabotaging her placements on purpose by breaking and destroying things; she was always hyperactive and angry. But this last time it was different. It really scared the foster mother. She is one of our good foster parents, she really tried to bond with this child, but Jessica destroyed things, threatened the foster mother, then packed her stuff and left the house! Then she said that a voice in her head told her to do it. She probably has schizophrenia like her bio mother. Are you going to keep her?"

INTRODUCTION

Emergency departments (EDs) are expected to evaluate patients rapidly and efficiently to assess their safety, diagnosis, and treatment needs.[1] However, there are many barriers to assessment, including individual and familial matters resulting in complex presentations, and systemic issues inherent within the ED, such as lack of information, lack of training of ED staff with regard to identifying and managing psychiatric illnesses, and scarce effective resources for inpatient or outpatient domains.[2] The high prevalence of traumatic events experienced by children and adolescents in the welfare system further muddies the clinical picture, leading to difficult diagnostic and disposition decisions (**Box 1**). This article endeavors to increase clinicians' understanding of child welfare–related issues and provides some insight toward tackling the challenges mentioned previously.

CHILDREN AND ADOLESCENTS IN CHILD WELFARE SYSTEMS

One in 25 children and adolescents interacts with the child welfare system each year,[3] either as a result of having their family investigated by child protective services, by receiving support services from a child welfare agency to prevent them from being removed from their home, or by being placed into foster care. One in 184 youth in the United States is living in foster care,[4] and 5.9% of youth will spend time in foster care at some point in their childhood (**Fig. 1**).[5]

Similar risk factors exist for those presenting to psychiatric ERs. Moreover, youth in foster care are more likely to have a mental disorder or substance use disorder than those who were never in foster care, and are 2.5 times more likely to seriously consider suicide and 4 times more likely to attempt suicide.[9–11] They are also 4 times more likely to be prescribed psychotropic medications, with 41.3% of those being prescribed medications receiving 3 or more classes of medication within the same month.[12]

Box 1
Key obstacles in the evaluation and management of welfare-involved children in the emergency department

Assessment stage:
- A lack of historical information
- A lack of collateral information (parents may be unavailable or uncooperative, caseworkers and others may not have complete information)

Diagnostic stage:
- A history of trauma complicates the diagnosis

Disposition stage:
- The instability of the situation complicates the decision: Where will the child go? What type of supervision will the child have? Who will follow-up with treatment?

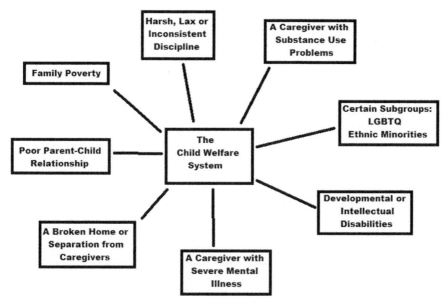

Fig. 1. Risk factors associated with entering the child welfare system. LGBTQ, lesbian, gay, bisexual, transgender, questioning or queer. (*Data from* Refs.[6–8])

The lack of preventive services, shortage of adequate intensive outpatient mental health resources,[2] and the lack of continuity of care due to relocation and change in foster care placement(s)[13] also often leads to ED presentations, whereas at other times, the ED visit itself generates the first encounter with the protective service agency as a result of a child's first disclosure of abuse or a caregiver refusing to pick up the child. It is important to remember that all physicians and all mental health practitioners are mandated reporters. That is, they are required by law to report, as soon as possible, any suspicion of child abuse or neglect, with civil and sometimes even criminal penalties being imposed against those who fail to report.[14]

TRAUMA AND CHILDREN AND ADOLESCENTS IN THE CHILD WELFARE SYSTEM

Traumatic events permeate the life of children and adolescents in the child welfare system. Their past experiences, the event that leads to the removal, the removal itself, and the secondary impacts of the removal, such as the uncertainty caused by chaotic and abrupt transitions (for example a change in living arrangement or school placement) can all be traumatizing.[15] Additionally, rates of abuse once in foster care are high, with studies suggesting that physical abuse is 3 times more likely and sexual abuse 2 to 4 times more likely in foster homes, and that physical abuse is 10 times more likely and sexual abuse 28 times more likely in group homes when compared with children not in foster care.[16]

Rates of previously traumatized youth visiting EDs are high and rates of youth engaged in the child welfare system are also elevated. Of 900 kids presenting to the Child Comprehensive Psychiatric Emergency Program at Bellevue Hospital in New York City, 51.7% responded positive to a pen and paper trauma screen, indicating experience with some type of prior abuse[17] and 36.1% of patients had current child welfare involvement (including those removed and those receiving preventive services).[17] Despite these numbers, trauma is often overlooked or ignored, and therefore, not considered when conducting an evaluation or when trying to understand the clinical picture, formulating diagnoses, or determining disposition.

LEGAL AND CONFIDENTIALITY-RELATED ISSUES

The clinical decisions of psychiatrists often affect their patients' civil liberties and, as such, more than any other medical specialty, the practice of psychiatry requires a familiarity with the laws relevant to the field. The legal issues involved become more complex when they pertain to minors and are complicated further still with respect to children in the welfare system. It should be noted that laws vary by jurisdiction, and discussion with a hospital attorney is recommended if there is any doubt about the applicable statute or legal standard in your area.

Often, the first issue to be addressed when a child presents to the ED is that of consent. Ordinarily, this is sought from the legal guardian of the child; in most cases the child's parent or parents. However, if parental rights have been surrendered or terminated or the child has been made free for adoption, the biological parents are no longer able to make decisions about the child. In such cases, the relevant foster care agency should be in possession of a court order giving them legal authority to make decisions on the child's behalf.[18] If parental rights have not been terminated, efforts should be made, and documented, to contact the parents to obtain informed consent for psychiatric evaluation and/or treatment of their child. If good faith efforts are made, but the parents either cannot be reached or are refusing to provide consent, there should be legal procedures in place to bypass or override this lack of consent if the evaluation and/or treatment is deemed to be clinically necessary, but efforts to obtain consent should continue after the emergent treatment has been provided. It should be noted that the person (caseworker, school or group home staff, foster parent) bringing the child to the ED often does not have the legal authority to make decisions for the child and the person may not even be aware of this. In such cases, a determination should be made as to who has this authority and efforts should be made to contact that person or organization.

There are many reasons that the biological parents of the child (assuming they still have legal custody despite not having physical custody) may not wish to consent to their child being psychiatrically evaluated or treated, including resistance to working with the agency, stigma, or misinformation and fears regarding mental health care in general or specifically regarding the agency wanting to "drug" their child. The conversation in the ED provides an opportunity to allay parental fears and improve engagement in their child's treatment,[19] which is especially important, as the ultimate goal of foster care is to reunite children with their families. Providing appropriate information about a child's need for psychiatric intervention and follow-up is invaluable in promoting the parent's continuous involvement with visitations and treatment, while empowering them to become an advocate for their child's needs.

Obtaining the necessary information about a child in an emergency is always challenging, but even more so when evaluating children involved with the child welfare system, as a result of the often chaotic and unpredictable life circumstances of such children. There are often various adults involved (biological parents, foster parents, foster agency staff, teachers, and medical and psychiatric providers), each of whom may have information from different stages of the child's life. Not only is the information from different adults prone to be contradictory and difficult to weave into a coherent narrative of the child's life, but there is the added complication of concerns about confidentiality. As the lives of these youth are often permeated with disruptions, constructing a timeline, especially in the context of identifying when symptoms have arisen, persisted, and/or escalated, is important (**Table 1**).

Table 1
Obtaining appropriate information from collateral sources

Whom to Contact?	What Information May They Know?
• Biological parent(s) if available	• Developmental history, early childhood history, past treatment history, family history
• Current foster parent(s) or adoptive parent(s)	• Recent behaviors, current function, and potential triggers
• Caseworker from protective agency or foster care agency (whose knowledge of the child/family will vary from having had one encounter, an emergency removal for example, to having worked with the family and child for a longer period)	• Reasons for the initial removal • Past documentation/evaluations, treatment history, current functioning, recent changes, and potential environmental stressors (such as changes in visitation status, lack of caregiver's involvement, foster parent's frustration level, and upcoming court hearings)
• School personnel (teacher[s], school counselor, school psychologist/social worker)	• Current academic and social functioning • Recent changes in behavior, mood, and attitude
• Current mental health providers	• Treatment course, response, and attendance • Clinical opinion

Because obtaining collateral information from various sources is necessary during an emergency evaluation, it is important to be aware of the rules regarding the disclosure and collection of information. Providers should make an attempt to obtain informed consent for seeking and providing information from other parties. If consent is not provided, then this exchange may occur under an "emergency exception" if such information is required to adequately perform the assessment, reach a diagnosis, and determine an appropriate disposition.[14]

PERFORMING A TRAUMA-INFORMED ASSESSMENT

After being asked: "What brought you here today?" Jessica responds with a long distant silence and a quick scan of the interview room. She adds: "Am I staying here?"

"Universal precautions" refer to general guidelines, followed by every single medical provider in every single encounter with a patient. Because welfare-involved youth presenting to an ED are highly likely to have experienced past traumatic events, providers in such a setting should adhere to "Universal Trauma Precautions," including developing rapport, remaining transparent about the process, and assessing trauma in a trauma-informed manner.[20] Consistent with the New Haven Trauma Competency,[21] such precautions are fundamental to the acts of gathering accurate information and understanding the youth's presentation in the larger context of past traumatic history, current stressors, and familial and environmental factors. Whether the presentation is indicative of trauma or not, a crucial step is to ask about a history of trauma, as most will not volunteer this information (**Table 2**).[21]

Table 2	
Factors making it difficult to speak about trauma	
Factors Making It Difficult for a Child to Speak with a Clinician About Trauma	**Factors Making It Difficult for a Clinician to Ask a Child About Trauma**
• Not being asked • Having received strong messages from adults in their lives to not talk about it or to "get over it" • Having been blamed for being a victim • Not having been believed once they disclosed previous trauma • Avoiding painful emotions and unpleasant thoughts related to the trauma • Not being aware that their trauma is related to what has been described as their "bad" or "crazy" behavior • Being afraid to "lose it" in the ED if triggered and subsequently being admitted or kept on a hold	• A lack of training in performing trauma-informed assessments • Personal discomfort (perhaps stemming from a personal history of trauma) • Not wanting to trigger or upset the youth • Not having enough time in an emergency department setting to ask in a sensitive manner • Lacking an awareness that trauma may contribute to the psychiatric presentation • Taking the child's initial "no" response at face value

Although the New Haven Trauma Competency and the 4 principles of "Universal Trauma Precautions" provide helpful evidence-based guidelines, they fail in providing concrete examples of the *"how to"* and *"what to"* ask for clinicians. Suggestions and examples are shared as follows[20]:

1. Developing rapport with clear and consistent boundaries.

    Being clear and direct about your role as the evaluator, your intent in performing the evaluation and the steps to be taken in your decision-making process, all while normalizing the youth's experience, is the first step to quickly creating rapport, decreasing the sense of helplessness, and increasing a sense of agency.

    Most kids who come in here ask me this… to be honest, I don't know yet… I'm going to try to get as much information as I can so we can make the best decision as a team. I'm going to speak with you while some of my colleagues are speaking with others who know you and might know what has been going on, so we can make the best recommendations to help you.

2. Explaining privacy and confidentiality.

    To get the best understanding of what is going on, we need to speak to those who know you well and who know what happened today. Other than your mother, foster mother, caseworker, and teacher, is there another adult who knows what's happening? By the way, I'm not telling them anything about you, I'm just trying to get information from them and from you to understand what's going on.

3. Systematically and repeatedly assessing trauma in a sympathetic way.

    The New Haven Trauma Competency reminds practitioners of the duty to ask about trauma while showing empathy and an ability to tolerate both the content and the affect presented by the individual.

    • Generalization:
        ○ "I'm going to ask you a bunch of questions that I ask all kids that I see, because a lot of us experience these things."
    • Explanation:
        ○ "I ask these questions because I want to make sure you are safe."

- Normalization:
  - "Lots of kids who are dealing with depression (or cutting themselves, or smoking weed a lot, or getting into fights) tell me that part of it is about dealing with (or escaping from) bad memories or painful feelings from things that have happened in the past."
  - "Most of the time, there is a good reason for a kid to miss school (or run away, cut, use drugs)...I wonder what's going on for you?"
- Validation:
  - "That must have been so hard/sad/confusing/frustrating."
- Empathy:
  - "I bet it hurts to talk or think about this."
  - "I can't imagine how it feels to go through all of this."
  - "It's so unfair that you had to go through that."
- Respecting avoidance:
  - "I get why you haven't talked about this."
  - "It makes sense you've been trying not to think about this—it sounds like it's just too hard."
- Showing respect:
  - "We don't have to talk about this anymore right now if you don't want to. If you need a break or want to come back to this another time that's cool, but I really want to make sure we talk about it because it's important to me to understand what you've been through."
- Using genuine praises:
  - "I know it's hard to talk about this. You are very strong for doing so and I'm really grateful that you're sharing it with me."
- Highlighting resiliency:
  - "You've been through so much, how have you been able to handle all of this?"
  - "Even with all of this, you've still been keeping up with school (or taking care of your siblings, or staying focused on your music or basketball)—how do you do that? Is there anyone who helps you or do you just do this on your own?"
- Expecting ambivalence:
  - "I can see how smoking weed (or cutting or running away or avoiding thinking about what happened) has helped you in dealing with all of this. Do you wish there were other ways to manage those painful memories (or thoughts or emotions)?"

Ask specifically, but start generally:

- *"Have you ever been through anything very scary? Like being part of or witnessing an accident? Violence in the neighborhood? Bullying at school?"*
- *"Has there been a time when you had to live apart from one of your parents?"*
- *"Have you ever lost someone close to you?"*
- *"Has anyone ever hit you? Or harmed you in other ways?"*
- *"Who yells the most in your house? Who fights in your house? Do the fights ever get physical?"*
- *"If you get in trouble at home, what happens as punishment?"*
- *"Has someone ever touched you inappropriately, or made you touch them in a way that made you uncomfortable?"*
- *"You mentioned you're dating someone. Does he treat you well? Has he ever threatened you? Hit you? Made you do anything sexually that you didn't want to do?"*
- *"Have you ever done sexual things in exchange for money/drugs/a place to stay?"*

4. Recognizing that an understanding of every child changes as more accurate information is provided by the collateral source(s), often when the child and other sources' trust in the evaluator increases.

Basic therapeutic skills, such as normalizing and validating (as described previously) in addition to asking about trauma often and considering gathering facts from a variety of sources is crucial. Building rapport and constructing an accurate timeline of events and surfacing of symptoms by obtaining information from multiple sources will allow for a more accurate diagnosis, which then informs appropriate recommendations and treatment.

BRINGING IT ALL TOGETHER: DECISIONS ABOUT DIAGNOSIS, DISPOSITION, AND TREATMENT
Challenges with Respect to Diagnosis and Treatment

Preparing an accurate and comprehensive biopsychosocial formulation may be an unattainable goal in the ED, but to ensure that our patients receive appropriate psychiatric care within the confines of an unfortunately imperfect and overburdened system it may be necessary to reach what at times is a difficult and unnerving compromise.[22] As discussed previously, children in the welfare system are more likely than other children to be diagnosed with a psychiatric disorder.[11] Given the almost ubiquitous presence of trauma in this population, it can be difficult to ascertain whether any of the psychiatric symptoms that are being seen or reported actually predated that trauma. Even if it can be clearly established that behavioral or emotional problems existed before trauma, it is likely that any subsequent trauma (including the trauma inherent in becoming involved in the welfare system) is contributing to or exacerbating the presentation. Keeping this in mind, it is important that as the evaluating clinician (and team), we do not add to this history of trauma. Tragically, children in the welfare system are all too used to hearing that they are "bad kids." The words and actions we use can influence (either positively or negatively) the way people talk to and about the child in the future, which can undoubtedly impact not only the child's view of themselves, but also how they are perceived and treated within the system. Identifying and focusing on a child's strengths and interests is an effective way not only to build rapport, but also to engender a sense of agency within the child and to provide focal points for encouraging their engagement.

If the child has preexisting psychiatric diagnoses, efforts should be made to confirm or refute those based on the currently available information, including being informed by a working knowledge of the approximate prevalence of certain psychiatric disorders in various age groups. For example, bipolar disorder is very uncommon in 6-year-olds; therefore, it is more likely that a history of disruptive, aggressive behavior and an irritable mood in a child in the welfare system is attributable to a trauma-related and stressor-related disorder, such as adjustment disorder or posttraumatic stress disorder. Taking into account the child's developmental stage and other factors, time should be spent on discussing diagnoses. This is an opportunity to provide some psychoeducation on the concept of trauma. While not endorsing any negative behaviors a child may have previously engaged in, it may be possible to validate the child's experience and to allow for the child (and the child's parents or other caregivers) to develop an understanding of the role of trauma in past behavioral issues.

The diagnosis that is reached should inform decisions about medications to be prescribed, adjusted, or discontinued. An ED evaluation is an opportunity to reassess the child's current medication regimen and, although it may not be practical to make changes in this setting, there is an opportunity to communicate with the child's prescriber any concerns and to give recommendations for adjustments, such as considering tapering off unhelpful and potentially harmful medications or optimizing regimens involving multiple medications. Particular care should be given to medications requiring close and regular monitoring (for example, of blood levels), as these children may be returning to potentially chaotic and unpredictable situations without the safety net of a predictable schedule or supervision.

When disposition recommendations include acute psychiatric hospitalization, state statutes regarding the procedural due process and substantive due process for psychiatric hospitalization must be met. These statutes vary by jurisdiction, and also with respect to whether the hospitalization is voluntary or involuntary. Additional protections also may be in place regarding the hospitalization of children in foster care.[13]

It should be noted that hospitalization should never be viewed as a "placement" to be used in the absence of available options within the welfare continuum. The purpose of the hospitalization should be explained to the child and the resulting feelings of rejection, not being wanted, or not being "good enough," should be explored and processed. There also should be an emphasis placed on visitation and the important role of parents or caregivers in the child's ongoing treatment.

If the child does not need psychiatric hospitalization, consideration should be given to the circumstances to which they will be discharged. (Return to a foster family with whom they are familiar, or an entirely new setting? If to a residential facility or group home, what is the level of staff supervision and training? Does the child already have outpatient psychiatric care in place or does the child need referral?)

The follow-up plan should be discussed with the child so that the child feels some sense of autonomy and has the opportunity to ask questions, but it must also be shared with the child's parents (if they are available) and members of agency staff that may be involved in coordinating such care.

Finally, clinicians should familiarize themselves with the trauma-informed mental health treatment options available in their area. The National Child Traumatic Stress Network provides a list of empirically based treatments for children and adolescents (http://nctsn.org/training-guidelines).[23]

After obtaining collateral information from various sources and using a trauma-informed approach while assessing Jessica, the clinical team explains to her caseworker and foster mother that Jessica's presentation meets criteria for an adjustment disorder with a differential diagnosis of posttraumatic stress disorder. This is received with some doubt from the caseworker who asks, "What about her hearing voices?" The clinical team provides psychoeducation from a biopsychosocial perspective about normal responses to trauma, early family disruptions, and constant fear of being rejected, leading to a better understanding of the diagnosis, disposition, and treatment recommendations, including deferring medications at this time. The foster mother is also able to better appreciate how Jessica's past experiences may be contributing to their interactions, especially as they have grown closer and as her mother's visits have become more inconsistent. After a brief family session, in the presence of the foster mother, the team assists with highlighting some of Jessica's strengths and addresses some of her fear resulting in the foster mother agreeing to take her home and participate in trauma-informed therapy on a weekly basis. The team also discusses a safety plan and strategies to be used by the foster mother should Jessica attempt to leave the house again. After more kind words are expressed back and forth between Jessica and her foster mother, Jessica turns to her foster mother and asks: "Do you think we can give horseback riding another try?" "Probably," answers the foster mother with a smile. "Let's talk about it when we get home."

The lives of children and adolescents in the child welfare system are often fragmented and misunderstood. A comprehensive and trauma-informed approach reconciles the full clinical picture, leads to a better understanding of presenting symptoms, highlights the child's strengths and improves caregivers' and providers' understanding and ability to care for these children.

REFERENCES

1. Zeller SL. Treatment of psychiatric patients in emergency settings. Prim Psychiatry 2010;17:41–7.
2. Hoyle JD, White LJ. Emergency Medical Services for Children; Health Resources Services Administration, Maternal and Child Health Bureau, National Association of EMS Physicians. Treatment of pediatric and adolescent mental health emergencies in the United States: current practices, models, barriers and potential solutions. Prehosp Emerg Care 2003;7:66–73.
3. Friedersdorf C. In a year, child-protective services checked up on 3.2 million children. The Atlantic. 2014. Available at: https://www.theatlantic.com/national/archive/2014/07/in-a-year-child-protective-services-conducted-32-million-investigations/374809/. Accessed October 3, 2017.
4. U.S. Department of Health and Human Services, Administration for children and families, administration on children, youth and families, children's bureau (2012). The AFCARS Report: preliminary FY 2011 estimates as of July 2012. Available at: http://www.acf.hhs.gov/sites/default/files/cb/afcarsreport19.pdf. Accessed October 3, 2017.
5. Wildeman C, Emanuel N. Cumulative risks of foster care placement by age 18 for U.S. children, 2000–2011. PLoS One 2014;9(3):e92785.
6. Park JM, Solomon P, Mandell DS. Involvement in the child welfare system among mothers with serious mental illness. Psychiatr Serv 2006;57(4):493–7.
7. Chaffin M, Kelleher K, Hollenberg J. Onset of physical abuse and neglect: psychiatric, substance abuse, and social risk factors from prospective community data. Child Abuse Neglect 1996;20(3):191–203.
8. Bowser BP, Jones T. Understanding the over-representation of African Americans in the child welfare system: San Francisco. Hayward (CA): The Urban Institute; 2004.
9. Pilowsky DJ, Wu LT. Psychiatric symptoms and substance use disorders in a nationally representative sample of American adolescents involved with foster care. J Adolesc Health 2006;38(4):351–8.
10. Pecora PJ, Romanelli LH, Jackson LJ, et al. Mental health services for children placed in foster care: an overview of current challenges. Child Welfare 2009;88(1):5–26.
11. Burns BJ, Phillips SD, Wagner HR, et al. Mental health needs and access to mental health services by youths involved with child welfare: a national survey. J Am Acad Child Adolesc Psychiatry 2004;43(8):960–70.
12. Zito JM, Safer DJ, Sai D, et al. Psychotropic medication patterns among youth in foster care. Pediatrics 2008;121(1):e157–63.
13. Rubin DM, Alessandrini EA, Feudtner C, et al. Placement stability and mental health costs for children in foster care. Pediatrics 2004;113(5):1336–41.
14. Fortunati FG Jr, Zonana HV. Legal considerations in the child psychiatric emergency department. Child Adolesc Psychiatr Clin N Am 2003;12:745–61.
15. American Academy of Pediatrics. Healthy Foster Care America. 2018. Available at: https://www.aap.org/en-us/advocacy-and-policy/aap-health-initiatives/healthy-foster-care-america/Pages/Mental-and-Behavioral-Health.aspx. Accessed October 3, 2017.

16. National Coalition for Child Protection Reform. Foster care vs. family prevention: the track record on safety and well being. Issue Paper 1. 2015. Available at: https://drive.google.com/file/d/0B291mw_hLAJsV1NUVGRVUmdyb28/view. Accessed March 5th, 2017.
17. Gerson R, Havens J, Marr M, et al. Utilization patterns at a specialized children's comprehensive psychiatric emergency program. Psychiatr Serv 2017;68(11): 1104–11.
18. Available at: https://www.nycourts.gov/courthelp/family/parentalRights.shtml. Accessed October 3, 2017.
19. Havens JF. Making psychiatric emergency services work better for children and families. J Am Acad Child Adolesc Psychiatry 2011;50(11):1093–4.
20. Gerson R, Heppell P. Beyond PTSD: helping and healing teens exposed to trauma. Arlington (VA): American Psychiatric Publishing, in press.
21. Cook JM, Newman E. A consensus statement on trauma mental health: The New Haven Competency Conference process and major findings. Psychological Trauma: Theory, Research, Practice, and Policy 2014;6(4):300–7. Available at: http://dx.doi.org/10.1037/a0036747. Accessed October 3, 2017.
22. Case SD, Case BG, Olfson M, et al. Length of stay in pediatric mental health emergency department visits in the United States. J Am Acad Child Adolesc Psychiatry 2011;50(11):1110–9.
23. National Child Traumatic Stress Network. National child traumatic stress network empirically supported treatments and promising practices. Available at: http://nctsn.org/training-guidelines. Accessed October 3, 2017.

Telepsychiatric Evaluation and Consultation in Emergency Care Settings

Austin Butterfield, MD

KEYWORDS

- Telepsychiatry • eMental health • Emergency psychiatry • Access to care
- Cost reduction

KEY POINTS

- New models of care and service delivery systems are needed to meet the mental health needs of youth in the setting of a worsening gap between available supply of qualified providers and demand for child psychiatric services.
- Telepsychiatry is a viable modality of care in the emergency setting with multiple established benefits including improving access to care and quality of care especially in underserved and rural areas and cost savings in a variety of contexts.
- Technological advances in video conferencing, security, confidentiality, and connection strength have improved the telepsychiatric experience for patients and clinicians.
- Telepsychiatric care in the emergency setting has become increasingly affordable and sustainable.
- Multiple models of telepsychiatric care around the world and within the United States demonstrate the flexibility of the technologies to meet highly variable needs in different regions.

INTRODUCTION

Various types of medical evaluations and treatments have been provided remotely using a variety of communication technologies for more than 70 years.[1] Psychiatry's history with remote care is among the longest of any specialty.[1] Widespread use of this modality of care delivery has become increasingly common around the world since the mid-1990s, and the rapid improvements in video quality and networking capabilities associated with the Internet and mobile technologies have significantly improved the viability of telepsychiatry as a modality of service delivery.[2,3]

No financial disclosures or conflicts of interests.
Department of Psychiatry, School of Medicine, University of Colorado, 13001 East 17th Place, Box F546, Aurora, CO 80045, USA
E-mail address: austin.butterfield@ucdenver.edu

Child Adolesc Psychiatric Clin N Am 27 (2018) 467–478
https://doi.org/10.1016/j.chc.2018.03.001
childpsych.theclinics.com

Telepsychiatry has been used in most clinical contexts including hospitals, emergency departments, and primary care for any mental health service (eg, diagnostic evaluations, medication management, consultation, psychotherapy), and data supporting telepsychiatric care as clinically effective and cost-efficient have increased over the past decade and a half.[4,5] Some of the previously theoretic advantages of telepsychiatric services, such as cost-savings and increased access to care, are now real-world benefits for the health care delivery systems that have embraced the new technologies and techniques.[6-9] Telepsychiatric care for emergencies has been more slowly adopted than for other clinical settings despite the increasing evidence for benefits and the well-documented increase nationally in emergency psychiatric visits.[4,6,10]

This article focuses on telepsychiatric care for children, teenagers, and their families in the emergency and urgent care contexts. The benefits, limitations, models, and strategies for implementation for emergency telepsychiatry are explored. Data for telepsychiatric emergencies with youth are particularly limited compared with adult literature and literature for other care settings (eg, primary care), but one consistent theme in literature relating to the use of telemental health services is that most data that support tele-encounters are generally similar in efficacy to standard face-to-face encounters in most contexts.[2,4,8] Experience with telepsychiatric services varies widely among child and adolescent psychiatrists (CAPs) and other mental health professionals. This article provides an accessible, user friendly overview and approach to this modality.

NATIONAL CRISIS CAUSED BY PSYCHIATRIC EMERGENCY VISITS

The national volume of children and adolescents visiting emergency rooms for psychiatric chief complaints has been increasing over multiple years.[10] The increased volume has overwhelmed available work force and resources in many communities. The national shortage of CAPs is well-documented, and the distribution of available CAPs is unequitable across the country.[11] Most CAPs live in major population centers, but most cities still have significantly fewer CAPs than necessary to address patient needs. The highly variable distribution of CAPs and other mental health professionals across the nation has intensified the challenges faced by many communities particularly in rural or other underserved areas.

Additionally, children seen with psychiatric emergencies and crises typically face longer wait times and higher admission rates than patients seen for medical-surgical issues and many patients in need of psychiatric hospitalization are required to wait in emergency departments for many hours or even weeks until an appropriate treatment setting is found.[12] By extension, "boarding," the practice of housing and treating patients with psychiatric emergencies in emergency departments when inpatient psychiatric hospital beds are unavailable, has become increasingly common for pediatric and adult patients.[13] The combination of all these factors has created what many consider to be a national crisis of care for evaluation and treatment of patients with psychiatric emergencies. Outcomes are often poor, and the crisis is costly for the limited financial and human resources.

COMMON LANGUAGE

Definitions related to technology in general and specifically referring to the integration of communication technologies and health services are a common source of confusion. New terms are frequently created and definitions of other terms drift over time. Although many definitions have not been fully standardized, the current discussion is consistent with the definitions provided in the American Telemedicine Association (ATA) glossary. A brief list of some helpful terms and synonyms is provided in **Table 1**. The ATA comprehensive glossary is available at their Web site (http://thesource.americantelemed.org/resources/telemedicine-glossary).

Table 1
Common terms related to telehealth

Term	Definition	Notes
Telehealth	Umbrella term for all health care services including nonclinical and nonmedical services provided through communication technologies	
Telemedicine	Term for any medical services provided remotely using communication technologies	Most often implies real-time video conferencing technologies as main mode of interaction
Telepsychiatry	A form of telemedicine that specifically relates to psychiatric services	
Telemental health	Umbrella term for any services for mental or behavioral health provided remotely using communication technologies	Includes services provided by nonmedically trained mental health providers (eg, licensed clinical social workers)
Originating site	Location of the patient or consulting provider receiving services by telecommunication technology	Synonyms: patient site, spoke site, remote site, rural site
Distant site	Location of physician or other licensed professional that provides services via telecommunication technology	Synonyms: physician/clinician site, hub site, specialty site, consulting site
Presenter	Person at originating site that manages the equipment and tasks that allow the patient to participate in the telehealth service	Synonyms: patient presenter • Legal and system-specific requirements for being a presenter may vary at organization, local, and state levels
Virtual private network	Method of securely using an Internet connection from a location outside an organization's location to access the benefits of a private network (eg, secure electronic medical record system, organization private files)	
Virtual desktop	Process of remotely connecting to a primary display screen (ie, desktop) for an organization to access files and programs securely	• Virtual desktop infrastructure is common form of virtual desktop in electronic medical record systems
Synchronous	Telehealth interaction that uses technology to allow communication between all parties at the same time	Synonyms: real-time • Usually uses videoconferencing or telephone
Asynchronous	Telehealth interaction that uses technology to provide communication between parties at different times	• Common examples are recorded videos and consultation reports (eg, radiology reports)

Prefixes: Tele-, e-, and m-

Prefixes added to disciplines and specialties are among the most confusing terms related to technology. Generally speaking, the prefix "e" is used for electronic and by extension can refer to any aspect of health care supported by electronically based technology (eg, patient portals, electronic medical records). The prefix "tele" refers to a subset of eHealth that uses video communication technology to provide health care services synchronously, as was the original use of the term "telepsychiatry" in the 1970s.[14] The prefix "m" is now most commonly used as a reference to mobile and portable technologies including smart phones and tablet computers that use applications (apps) to provide services or support. m-Mental health options tend to be more varied for context and purpose than telemental health because the mobile devices are by nature portable. The applications also allow for synchronous (eg, videoconferencing with therapist) and asynchronous services (eg, recording of mindfulness exercise). Because the mobile technologies are newer than other communication technologies, less data are currently available for their clinical use. However, emerging evidence is encouraging for their potential efficacy in treating various mental health conditions and for connecting families, patients, and providers.[7]

All the previously mentioned prefixes refer only to the application of the technology as part of care. None of the prefixes indicate a specific discipline, specialty, or subspecialty currently. A Venn diagram demonstrating the overlap of some commonly used terms with the tele-prefix is provided in **Fig. 1**. The relations presented with the tele-prefix in the Venn diagram are interchangeable with e- and m-prefixes as descriptions of the relationships (eg, m-mental health falls as a subset of m-health).

RATIONALE FOR TELEPSYCHIATRY IN EMERGENCY SETTINGS

Communities and systems of care around the country have approached the crisis created by increasing mental health visits in emergency rooms in a variety of ways, but telepsychiatry has been increasingly seen as one of the key strategies to better address the needs of these patients and families. The evidence base for benefits of telepsychiatry outside the emergency setting is already robust.[5]

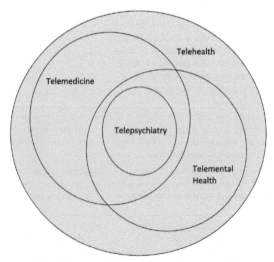

Fig. 1. Venn diagram of disciplines and specialties with tele-prefix.

Benefits of telepsychiatry in different settings include increased access to care, high satisfaction levels of patients and providers, and statistically equivalent outcomes compared with face-to-face care in most studies.[3,5,15] Improvement for access to care for underserved communities and regions has been one of the most commonly cited benefits of telepsychiatric care.[8,11,16] Telepsychiatry allows a variety of services to be offered in rural and other underserved areas that would otherwise be unavailable.[11,17] Other potential benefits in acute care settings include

- Decreased rates of unnecessary hospitalizations
- Potentially reduced lengths of hospitalization for patients requiring acute hospitalization
- Decreased wait times for evaluations
- Improved use of limited space and resources in general emergency departments
- Decreased length of stay in emergency departments
- Increased connection to outpatient resources
- Varying degrees of cost savings
- Higher quality of care in rural and underserved regions
- Decreased travel costs for patients and mental health professionals
- Improved experiences for patients and families

Because of the significant limitations of data available specifically for telepsychiatric emergency care currently, studies for pediatric and adult populations are explored next. Although the results of programs focused on adult populations are not automatically generalizable to pediatric populations, they are encouraging for psychiatric emergency care in general. Additionally, some health systems described next use this modality for psychiatric emergencies across the life span.

RECENT OUTCOME DATA HIGHLIGHTS FOR TELEPSYCHIATRIC EMERGENCY CARE

In South Carolina, Narasimhan and colleagues[18] described a state-wide telepsychiatric consultation service and compared several outcome measures for a large number of adult patients (7261 patients receiving telepsychiatric care, 7261 matched control subjects without telepsychiatric intervention, and 1805 patients who received telepsychiatric care without specific matched control subjects) over about 4 years. Outcome measures included hospitalization rates, lengths of hospitalizations for patients admitted after the emergency visit, follow-up rates in the outpatient setting, costs for the inpatient stays, and total costs. Patients were less likely to be admitted psychiatrically if the telepsychiatric service was used, and the overall length of stay of psychiatric hospitalizations for those who were admitted was statistically shorter for patients receiving telepsychiatric intervention versus care as usual. Their data unsurprisingly supported lower costs associated with inpatient hospitalizations, but they did not find statistically different costs at 30 days after the emergency department visit. Additionally, their analysis showed significantly increased follow-up with outpatient resources because of improved care coordination.

Southard and colleagues[19] explored the impact of telepsychiatric care in rural Indiana. Their team completed a retrospective chart review of 62 patients with comparisons of different measures before and after implementing a telepsychiatric consultation program for a rural hospital emergency department including pediatric patients. Time to order of consultation, time to evaluation, and length of stay in the emergency departments significantly decreased after the implementation of the telepsychiatric system. The changes in hospital policies after the implementation of the telepsychiatry consultation service contributed to the decrease in mean time results.

The availability of consultation expanded to 24-hours per day and the hospital also changed the policy of admitting patients for observation. Before the implementation of the telepsychiatry consultation model, all patients were admitted for observation, but the hospital allowed for discharge after evaluation following the implementation of the telepsychiatry service. This mostly impacted mean length of stay. The secondary benefit of decreased transit times for the evaluators that would have to drive large distances was discussed, but no data were provided regarding specific cost or time savings to the clinicians. Despite limitations of study design with confounding policy factors and few patients, these additional data in the context of the growing body of literature continue to support the beneficial impact of telepsychiatry on care delivery systems.

Children's Hospital Colorado (the author's home institution) also has recently published data on the ongoing use of telepsychiatric care in the pediatric emergency department. Thomas and colleagues[9] explored the impact of the implementation of a telepsychiatric consultation service for multiple emergency and urgent care locations in a large hospital system across the greater Denver-Aurora metropolitan area in Colorado. Outcome measures included length of stay in the emergency setting, disposition type, and hospital charges. These were analyzed before and after the implementation of the telepsychiatric consultation service. The addition of the telepsychiatric consultation option was associated with significantly decreased average lengths of stay in the emergency and urgent care locations. This study also showed that the use of telepsychiatric consultations significantly decreased average total patient charges for the emergency visit by an average of more than $5000 compared with care as usual. As has been found in other treatment contexts and studies, survey data collected as part of the project showed that patients, parents/guardians, and primary emergency providers were all highly satisfied with the process of the videoconferencing consultation. In the survey data, families often wrote statements of appreciation for avoiding ambulance transfers to the main Children's Hospital Colorado campus. The decrease in ambulance transfers contributed to the results demonstrating the model of consultation as cost-efficient for the hospital system.

PEDIATRIC EMERGENCY TELEMENTAL HEALTH MODELS

Traditionally, many emergency departments without specific mental health providers partnered with local mental health centers to provide on-call psychiatrists or other mental health clinicians. In rural and underserved areas in particular, these arrangements combined with low availability of the resources contributed to long wait-times, delays of appropriate disposition, and emergency room overcrowding. The mental health provider would be required go to the emergency department to complete the evaluation. Many current models of providing emergency telemental health care are adaptations of current in-person, standard-of-care evaluations rather than new techniques designed specifically around the technology. Several proof-of-concept and program evaluation studies for emergency telemental health and telepsychiatry have been published in the United States and other countries.[9,16,18–20]

Models of telemental health care are categorized by different characteristics including defined roles of team members (eg, direct patient care vs provider consultation without direct patient care) and timing (real-time video conferencing vs review of recorded material).[14,15,21,22] Additionally, emergency departments can hire internal providers to complete evaluations or partner with other organizations or individuals to obtain the services. Larger systems of care with multiple sites often have their own internally hired mental health providers, which can have benefits for space saving, centralization of resources, and decrease in time measures in emergency departments throughout the system. Partnerships with external mental health systems can provide similar benefits for emergency departments and hospitals that would not be able to financially sustain internally hired mental health providers.

Given the severe shortage of all mental health providers, multiple disciplines are used in different models of telemental health. Psychiatrists, psychologists, physician assistants, advance practice nurses, and clinical social workers can have different roles.[23] Depending on the available resources and specific goals of the telemental health program, a variety of multidisciplinary approaches can meet patient and family care needs. For example, clinical social workers evaluated patients via videoconferencing and then reviewed the cases with a CAP in the model for Children's Hospital Colorado described in the previous section.[9]

The availability of different models creates opportunities for customization of services to best fit the needs of patients and families served by different institutions. Given the nature of emergency settings, most models have emphasized improving the speed of appropriate evaluation, treatment recommendations, and disposition plan. Many emergency departments have opted for synchronous (ie, real-time), direct evaluations via videoconferencing by the telemental health provider.

TIPS AND STRATEGIES FOR CREATING AN EMERGENCY TELEMENTAL HEALTH SERVICE

Multiple organizations and experts have provided guidelines and considerations for designing and implementing telemental health services over the past decade.[2,8,11,15,22,23] Lessons have also been learned from proof-of-concept publications.[16,18] For those with backgrounds in quality improvement strategies or educational curriculum design models, the recommendations for starting telepsychiatric programs sound familiar. Common themes among recommendations include performing community needs assessments, identifying specific patient populations, evaluating current available resources in an area, designing model before implementation, ensuring appropriate technological infrastructure, and creating a process for program re-evaluation.[9,11,22–24] A variety of high-quality checklists and guidelines have been proposed since initial theoretic guidelines by Shore and colleagues[21] in 2007.[8,9,11,23,25] The ATA, the Academy of Child and Adolescent Psychiatry, and other national organizations have been building online resources and guidelines for potential programs. For the purposes of the current article, a stepwise approach adapted from the previously mentioned sources and lessons from a variety of programs is presented in **Box 1**.

Needs Assessment Phase

A needs assessment helps establish the goals of any program to match the needs of a potential patient population and necessary services. A needs assessment often includes gathering information about the current state of care provided in a system or region and the resources available to meet the current demand. Additionally, the needs assessment specifically identifies stakeholders and provides information about a potential target population. Without this initial information, the subsequent stages of program design are generally not possible.

For example, if a rural community hospital emergency department averages one psychiatric emergency visit every week, a full telepsychiatric service developed by the hospital may be unsustainable financially. However, this emergency department may find that contracting with another organization that provides telepsychiatric services to many hospitals in their state would be cost-efficient and improve care

---

Box 1
Stepwise approach for emergency telemental health program design

1. Needs assessment phase
   a. Evaluation of current state of care and resources
   b. Evaluation of current demand for service
   c. Survey of identified patient population
   d. Survey of potential providers
   e. Identification of potential barriers

2. Financial planning phase
   a. Cost-benefit analysis
   b. Financial model design (eg, provider fee-for-service, department funded, grant funded)
   c. Contract negotiations between organizations if needed
   d. Grant applications if available
   e. Malpractice coverage for all providers
   f. Obtain any needed support of senior administrators

3. Model design phase
   a. Set goals around specific needs of identified population
   b. Design parameters to measure of success/impact toward specified goals
   c. Decide scope of service based on financial data and obtainable resources
   d. Standardization of expected credentialing and licensing requirements to match state and local regulations
   e. Workflow design (eg, check-in procedure, process of starting consultation)
   f. Definition of roles for team members (eg, providers, information technology support, operations manager)
   g. Clarification of technical and clinical needs at originating site (ie, site of patient) and distant site (ie, site of provider)
   h. Identify space needs at both sites

4. Set-up phase
   a. Purchase of any needed technology or software licenses (eg, HIPPA-compliant videoconferencing service)
   b. Obtain any needed licensing
   c. Education and training for providers including billing codes and best practices for patient interactions
   d. Education and training for all nonprovider team members at both sites
   e. Practice runs of workflow and trouble-shooting
   f. Optimize telehealth rooms at both sites (eg, size, seating, lighting, camera location, color scheme)

5. Implementation phase
   a. Pilot program
   b. Start data collection for set parameters
   c. Re-evaluation with full implementation

6. Re-evaluation and quality improvement cycle phase
   a. Ongoing data collection
   b. Systematic program updates (eg, technological advancements, practice parameter changes)

---

provided. Major systems of care that have multiple satellite locations in a region may find that an internal telemental health service would best meet the needs of patients and families.

Financial Planning and Model Design Phases

Financial planning and model design are distinct, but related phases of development. Although both are essential, starting with a cost-benefit analysis of potential telemental health programs may allow better understanding of feasibility of a variety of models. Ideal care models are often not feasible because of initial financial constraints, but in some communities or regions any level of new psychiatric emergency care service may represent a significant improvement.[9,22]

Regulatory and administrative issues become important considerations during the financial planning and model design phases.[21,26] Challenges are technical, clinical, legal, or ethical. For example, credentialing and documentation privileges are obstacles when the telemental health services are contracted between different organizations. Similarly, state licensing is a barrier to improving access in underserved regions in the setting of the previously discussed inequitable distribution of mental health resources.[8,11,21] Providers generally must be licensed in the state where the patient will be treated. This is expensive for providers, although there have been many calls for updating of licensing regulations to better allow providers to meet the needs of patients and families across state lines.[8] Ensuring that a process is created for providers to comply with local and state laws of the originating site is essential.

All programs need specific and measurable goals based on the information obtained in the needs assessment. Examples of goals for emergency telepsychiatric programs include decreased wait-times to be seen, decreased time to the appropriate disposition plans, and improved patient satisfaction with services provided. Establishing the specific goals while designing the system is important to ensure that data are collected and the program's results and impact re-evaluated over time to meet the changing needs of patients and families after implementation.

Set-Up Phase

After a program has been designed, additional training and education is typically needed for all team members involved at all sites including providers, nurses, support staff, administrators, and information technology personnel. Education needs often include understanding the available hardware (eg, cameras), software, the designed workflow, billing (if present), and specific roles for each team members. Although security of technology has continually improved, legal and ethical considerations of privacy remain paramount. Adequate sound reduction at the physical sites is an issue and should be considered when establishing the space for patients and providers. Additionally, a variety of videoconferencing programs are available that meet HIPPA standards. Integration of videoconferencing programs and electronic medical records is challenging. Working with the identified information technology support personnel can improve the experience of users across the different programs.

Anecdotally, the videoconferencing capabilities are used for relationship and trust building between team members at the different sites. Having a good baseline relationship between the sites is important. At the author's home institution, relationship building has been helpful in reducing conflicts during high-stress patient encounters that are common in the emergency setting. As such, trust and relationship building exercises between different team members is recommended during this phase.

Much has been written about telehealth etiquette (general considerations for improved social interactions while videoconferencing). Some aspects of telehealth etiquette are addressed by optimization of the physical space and technology. A common example of this is minimization of the angle between the camera and screen to allow better approximation of eye contact.[2,11,26,27] Some aspects of telehealth etiquette are slight modifications in interview style on the part of the provider, such as the use of more expressive or energetic communication style, introduction of all participants in the room, and allowing patients to consent or assent to the parties present in the rooms.[26] Educating team members and subsequently patients and families on process and etiquette can improve overall satisfaction with the process.

Implementation Phase, Re-evaluation Process, and Quality Improvement Cycle

The implementation stage of the process is the most straightforward. Many choose to implement the process as a pilot program with a limited time frame before re-evaluation of some key measures to make sure that the goals of the program are specifically being addressed by the current design. Modifications and updates to policies and procedures after the pilot program can often be quickly implemented. However, data collection and re-evaluation of goals of the telemental health program remain crucial, given that technology and best practices in the setting are not fully established.

SUMMARY

As the number of psychiatric emergency visits continues to increase for all age groups, telepsychiatry in the emergency setting will become more common and popular. Advances in the technologies used to provide this type of service continue to improve in quality and decrease in cost. At this point, continuing to use best practices adapted from face-to-face encounters is the standard for telemental health evaluations. However, significantly more data are needed to start establishing best practices specific to telepsychiatry in general.

Given that the currently available data for emergency telepsychiatry are limited but overall positive, increasing the number of programs that are participating in data collection in different contexts will be important in the coming years. Impacts on patient wait-times, boarding in emergency departments, and number of unnecessary hospitalizations are all part of the conversation. Further optimization is needed in many clinical situations including for different populations (eg, rural vs underserved urban areas), for different clinical presentations (eg, teenagers with suicidality vs first presentation of mania in a rural area), and for translation services. As the modality continues to increase in popularity, educational and training models for different disciplines will require updates, and integration into general residency and child and adolescent fellowship programs will be essential for preparing trainees for future career needs.[25]

Increased use of the modality may have less obvious benefits that should also be studied. For example, the decreased amount of driving by providers and patients could have cost-efficiencies for traffic flow, carbon emissions, and wear-and-tear on vehicles. Organizations that previously sent clinicians to different sites over large geographic areas may save money by decreasing mileage reimbursement.

Governments at the federal, state, and local levels across the country are adapting at different rates to the ongoing and rapid technological information evolutions. Outdated regulations are barriers to care as discussed in the previously mentioned implementation model. However, the combination of data for direct benefits to patients, cost-savings for health care systems, and secondary benefits (eg, decreased traffic) could be used to help shape public policy.

REFERENCES

1. Zundel KM. Telemedicine: history, applications, and impact on librarianship. Bull Med Libr Assoc 1996;84(1):71–9.
2. Gloff NE, LeNoue SR, Novins DK, et al. Telemental health for children and adolescents. Int Rev Psychiatry 2015;27(6):513–24.

3. Salmoiraghi A, Hussain S. A systematic review of the use of telepsychiatry in acute settings. J Psychiatr Pract 2015;21(5):389–93.
4. Hilty DM, Ferrer DC, Parish MB, et al. The effectiveness of telemental health: a 2013 review. Telemed J E Health 2013;19(6):444–54.
5. Hubley S, Lynch SB, Schneck C, et al. Review of key telepsychiatry outcomes. World J Psychiatry 2016;6(2):269–82.
6. Letvak S, Rhew D. Assuring quality health care in the emergency department. Healthcare (Basel) 2015;3(3):726–32.
7. Hilty DM, Chan S, Hwang T, et al. Advances in mobile mental health: opportunities and implications for the spectrum of e-mental health services. Mhealth 2017;3:34.
8. Myers K, Nelson EL, Rabinowitz T, et al. American telemedicine association practice guidelines for telemental health with children and adolescents. Telemed J E Health 2017;23(10):779–804.
9. Thomas JF, Novins DK, Hosokawa PW, et al. The use of telepsychiatry to provide cost-efficient care during pediatric mental health emergencies. Psychiatr Serv 2018;69(2):161–8.
10. Carubia B, Becker A, Levine BH. Child psychiatric emergencies: updates on trends, clinical care, and practice challenges. Curr Psychiatry Rep 2016; 18(4):41.
11. American Academy of Child and Adolescent Psychiatry (AACAP) Committee on Telepsychiatry and AACAP Committee on Quality Issues. Clinical update: telepsychiatry with children and adolescents. J Am Acad Child Adolesc Psychiatry 2017;56(10):875–93.
12. Dolan MA, Fein JA, Committee on Pediatric Emergency Medicine. Pediatric and adolescent mental health emergencies in the emergency medical services system. Pediatrics 2011;127(5):e1356–66.
13. Hazen EP, Prager LM. A quiet crisis: pediatric patients waiting for inpatient psychiatric care. J Am Acad Child Adolesc Psychiatry 2017;56(8):631–3.
14. Comer JS, Myers K. Future directions in the use of telemental health to improve the accessibility and quality of children's mental health services. J Child Adolesc Psychopharmacol 2016;26(3):296–300.
15. Shore J. The evolution and history of telepsychiatry and its impact on psychiatric care: current implications for psychiatrists and psychiatric organizations. Int Rev Psychiatry 2015;27(6):469–75.
16. Saurman E, Johnston J, Hindman J, et al. A transferable telepsychiatry model for improving access to emergency mental health care. J Telemed Telecare 2014; 20(7):391–9.
17. Rachal J, Sparks W, Zazzaro C, et al. Highlight in telepsychiatry and behavioral health emergencies. Psychiatr Clin North Am 2017;40(3):585–96.
18. Narasimhan M, Druss BG, Hockenberry JM, et al. Impact of a telepsychiatry program at emergency departments statewide on the quality, utilization, and costs of mental health services. Psychiatr Serv 2015;66(11):1167–72.
19. Southard EP, Neufeld JD, Laws S. Telemental health evaluations enhance access and efficiency in a critical access hospital emergency department. Telemed J E Health 2014;20(7):664–8.
20. Roberts N, Hu T, Axas N, et al. Child and adolescent emergency and urgent mental health delivery through telepsychiatry: 12-month prospective study. Telemed J E Health 2017;23(10):842–6.
21. Shore JH, Hilty DM, Yellowlees P. Emergency management guidelines for telepsychiatry. Gen Hosp Psychiatry 2007;29(3):199–206.

22. Yellowlees P, Burke MM, Marks SL, et al. Emergency telepsychiatry. J Telemed Telecare 2008;14(6):277–81.
23. Olson CA, Thomas JF. Telehealth: no longer an idea for the future. Adv Pediatr 2017;64(1):347–70.
24. Myers KM, Valentine JM, Melzer SM. Feasibility, acceptability, and sustainability of telepsychiatry for children and adolescents. Psychiatr Serv 2007;58(11): 1493–6.
25. Nelson EL, Cain S, Sharp S. Considerations for conducting telemental health with children and adolescents. Child Adolesc Psychiatr Clin N Am 2017;26(1):77–91.
26. Shore JH. Telepsychiatry: videoconferencing in the delivery of psychiatric care. Am J Psychiatry 2013;170(3):256–62.
27. Sorvaniemi M, Santamäki O. Telepsychiatry in emergency consultations. J Telemed Telecare 2002;8(3):183–4.

Psychiatric Community Crisis Services for Youth

Kristina Sowar, MD[a],*, Deborah Thurber, MD[b], Jeffrey J. Vanderploeg, PhD[c],
Eva C. Haldane, PhD[c]

KEYWORDS

- Community • Child • Family • Psychiatry • Crisis • Emergency • Services
- Interventions

KEY POINTS

- Epidemiologic data reflect increasing numbers of children and families presenting to emergency services for psychiatric care; however, standard emergency departments are often under-resourced to effectively meet their needs.
- A variety of care models have been devised to better support youths and families in psychiatric crises; these include mobile crisis services, phone triage lines, and observation and brief residential services.
- Key tenets to implementing such services include coordination with community stakeholders, leverage and collaboration with existing agencies, assessment and application for funding sources, evaluation and education around staffing needs, and continued quality improvement.
- Data reflect improved outcomes clinically and financially when communities implement a continuum of crises services.

INTRODUCTION

Children and families are seeking behavioral health care in record numbers, often with severe symptoms, including suicidal ideation, aggression, high risk–taking behaviors, and psychosis. In most communities, children and families in crisis present to emergency departments (EDs), which are often ill prepared and/or underequipped to provide adequate psychiatric evaluation, stabilization, and discharge planning. Given the challenges faced by our traditional medical systems in meeting these needs, communities can greatly benefit from developing and expanding psychiatric crisis care services for youths and families.

Disclosure Statement: No financial interests to disclose.
[a] Department of Child and Adolescent Psychiatry, University of New Mexico, 1001 Yale Boulevard Northeast, Albuquerque, NM 87131, USA; [b] Youth and Family Services, Ventura County Behavioral Health, 1911 Williams, Oxnard, CA 93036, USA; [c] Child Health and Development Institute of Connecticut, Inc, 270 Farmington Avenue, Suite 367, Farmington, CT 06032, USA
* Corresponding author.
E-mail address: ksowar@salud.unm.edu

Child Adolesc Psychiatric Clin N Am 27 (2018) 479–490
https://doi.org/10.1016/j.chc.2018.03.002
1056-4993/18/© 2018 Elsevier Inc. All rights reserved.

In this article, the authors highlight 2 crisis care models that have been successfully implemented at the community and state level. The authors review the development, implementation, as well as the clinical and financial outcomes of these models.

Data reflect what many health providers anecdotally observe: a continuous increase in children and families seeking care for psychiatric crises, including suicidal ideation, aggression, psychosis, substance intoxication, and severe family conflict. National data between 2006 and 2011 indicate a 50% increase in hospital admissions for mental health conditions, a 21% increase in ED visits for primary psychiatric concerns in children 10 to 14 years old, and a total of $11.6 billion spent on mental health in hospital settings during this time frame.[1] With nationwide shortages of child psychiatric providers (particularly in rural and poor, urban areas[2]), a decrease in number and availability of inpatient and residential beds, and insufficiently developed community-based treatment systems, children and families often face limited options for crisis care outside of standard emergency services.[3] Unfortunately, EDs often lack appropriate space and/or professionals with psychiatric training; so youths and families often face long wait times and limited options for intervention and follow-up. Children who are directed to inpatient admission may spend days boarding in EDs and inpatient medical floors, which occupies prized medical space and can be disruptive and stressful for youths and families.[1] Furthermore, there is limited evidence that inpatient treatment is the most effective treatment of many conditions, such as conduct disorder; other models of care are more effective for many children and families.[3] With these considerations in mind, it is clear that thinking outside the box to consider a continuum of crisis care services can better meet community needs.

The Substance Abuse and Mental Health Services Administration (SAMHSA) defines crisis services as a "continuum of services provided to individuals who experience a psychiatric emergency, with goals of stabilizing and improving psychological symptoms of distress, and engaging individuals in an appropriate treatment service to address the problem that led to the crisis."[4] Crisis services generally involve screening, evaluation and risk assessment, brief solution-focused interventions, and referral and linkage to ongoing care. Many communities have adult crisis services, such as assertive community treatment and crisis intervention teams, which engage with individuals in their community setting and interface with law enforcement to provide care; however, such services are less prevalent for children and adolescents.[4]

Additional examples of core crisis services include phone triage and warm lines that help with assessment and referral of youths to appropriate services; mobile crisis units that "go out into the community to begin the process of assignment and definitive treatment outside of a hospital or health care facility";[4] and psychiatric teams embedded within EDs that respond to psychiatric needs or incorporate short-term observation and residential beds.[4]

Several communities have implemented psychiatric crisis services for youths; this article describes the development and integration of programs in Ventura County, California and in Connecticut. The development and implementation of these crisis services share several themes: teamwork with community stakeholders; leverage and development of current services; expanded hiring and training for staff; and ongoing evaluation and collection of outcome measures, including psychiatric admission rate, repeated use of the ED, and linkage to ongoing treatment.

The Ventura County Non–Hospital-Based Continuum of Care Model for Youths in Mental Health Crisis

Ventura County, California is situated along the Pacific Coast between Los Angeles and Santa Barbara counties; it has a population of approximately 850,000.[5] Ventura

County Behavioral Health (VCBH) is the primary public mental health agency in this county, serving youths and adults with serious emotional and behavioral dysfunction and substance use disorders.

Overview

In 2014, county mental health providers and advocates raised formal concerns about increasingly limited local options for assessment, referral, and stabilization of youths in mental health crisis, leading to overuse of local EDs as interim placements. These concerns were evidenced by data: within the preceding 3 years, there had been a dramatic increase (68%) in calls, 43% increase in involuntary holds, and a 37% increase in psychiatric hospitalizations fielded by the countywide, mobile Children's Intensive Response Team. The county's only psychiatric hospital for youths was often full, as were other hospitals statewide, so many children were admitted far from home. At times, the Ventura County Adult Inpatient Unit would temporarily house youths until an adolescent bed opened; however, they soon ceased this practice, as they were not clinically licensed or equipped to handle this population, which led to further ED backups.

To better meet the community's burgeoning mental health needs, a Children's Crisis Task Force was developed. Stakeholders included individuals from the public health system, EDs, juvenile probation, child welfare, law enforcement, and mental health treatment agencies. The task force's mission was to evaluate best practices for youths in mental health crises and devise recommendations for a countywide continuum of care services. The task force embraced services as a mobile mental health crisis team, short-term crisis and residential units, and a community aftercare team to ensure connection with services. VCBH was charged with implementation of the model, either directly or through contractual arrangements with other clinical organizations (**Fig. 1**).

The VCBH clinical administrative team toured several programs that provided innovative crisis services for inspiration and examples; they decided to contract with a locally based nonprofit agency (Seneca) that had experience providing a youth mobile crisis response team, partial hospitalization, one-to-one intensive stabilization services, and short-term crisis residential programs. The County Board of Supervisors supported the purchase and remodeling of facilities to house the services.

Clinical staff were hired and trained and connected with county leadership to develop assessment and treatment protocols and procedures. This process involved multiple meetings to assure clear communication, definitions of roles and responsibilities, and seamless transitions of youths through the continuum of services. Specific flow charts were developed to assist EDs, schools, and group homes on protocols for accessing crisis services. A checklist was devised to help ED staff and first responders determine if a youth would need medical screening before admission to the psychiatric services. VCBH also expanded and retrained their existing adult mobile crisis team to include youth services.

Program Details

The Ventura County Children's Crisis Continuum consists of 4 main components: a 24/7 mobile VCBH crisis team, the less than 24-hour crisis stabilization unit (CSU), the short-term crisis residential team (CRT), and aftercare and connection to outpatient mental health services and other local resources through the VCBH Rapid Integrated Support and Engagement (RISE) Team (**Fig. 2**).

The Ventura County Mobile Crisis Team provides 24/7 crisis intervention, stabilization, and evaluation for county residents of all ages, regardless of

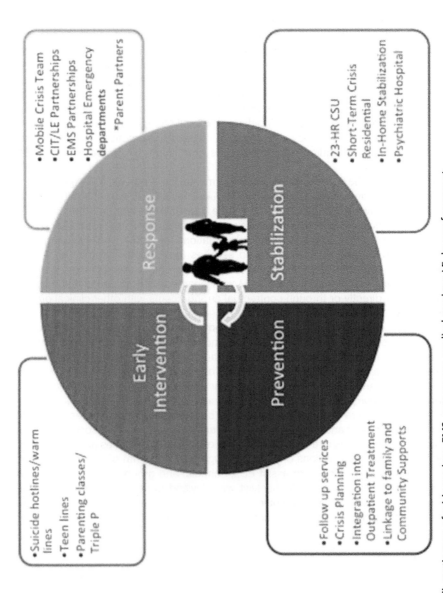

Fig. 1. Ideal full continuum of crisis services. EMS, emergency medical services; LE, law enforcement.

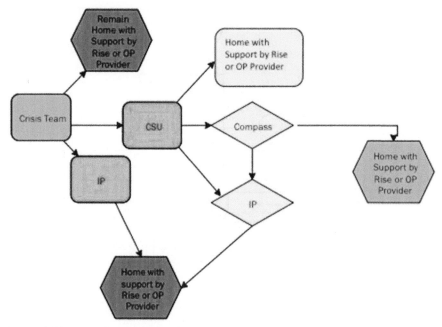

Fig. 2. Children's crisis continuum of care. IP, inpatient; OP, outpatient.

insurance status. Patients can be referred to higher levels of care when indicated. Goals for the mobile crisis team are to deescalate mental health crises and use tools to help youths remain at home/in the community, including safety planning and connecting families to resources and mental health services. The mobile crisis team can respond to any setting, including residences, schools, EDs, mental health and ambulatory care clinics, and Juvenile Hall. Staff represent many disciplines, including social workers, family therapists, nurses, and psychiatric technicians, and often respond to crises in pairs. They are supervised and supported by 2 program-specific administrators. The mobile crisis team is funded through a combination of direct billing to MediCal (California Medicaid) or private insurance, funds from the California Mental Health Services Act (MHSA), and state sales tax.

The CSU provides assessment, stabilization, and referral to mental health services for Ventura County youths ages 6 to 17 years, regardless of insurance status. It is licensed as a less than 24-hour, unlocked, 4-bed outpatient facility; youths can be accepted on a voluntary or involuntary basis. CSU is staffed by a multitude of providers, including masters' level clinicians, nurses, mental health counselors and child and adolescent tele-psychiatrists. Youths are assessed to determine if they can be stabilized enough to return home or require transfer to the CRT or inpatient psychiatric hospital for further intensive treatment. The goal of CSU treatment is to help youths and caregivers stabilize from acute crisis, develop a safety plan, and link with outpatient mental health providers. Direct billing to MediCal provides funding for services, supplemented by MHSA and the state sales tax fund (and possibly state funds in the future) (**Figs. 3** and **4**).

The Short-Term Crisis Stabilization Unit, called COMPASS, is an unlocked facility that serves up to 2 youths aged 12 to 17 years who are initially admitted to the CSU

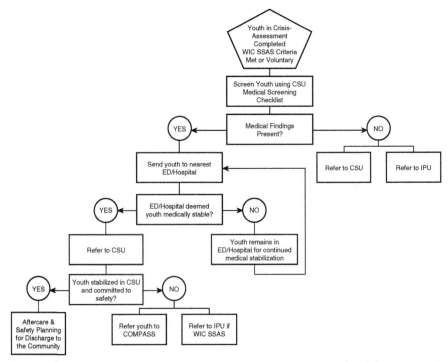

Fig. 3. Referral flow chart. COMPASS, Comprehensive Assessment and Stabilizaton Servcie (short term residential for Medi-Cal youth 12–17); CSU, VCBH Crisis Stabilization Unit-psychiatric treatment for youth 6–17 (regardless of insurance); ED, emergency department; Findings, medical findings based on checklists; IPU, inpatient psychiatric unit; VCBH, Ventura County Behavioral Health.

but require further stabilization and treatment services before returning home. Like the CSU, a multidisciplinary team staffs COMPASS; a tele-psychiatrist provides psychiatric assessment and follow-up for youths and consults with the treatment team, manages medication, and collaborates with outpatient mental health providers. While on the COMPASS unit, youths also receive intensive individual and family therapy, case management, and referral to aftercare services. An onsite teacher, funded by the county school districts, provides for temporary educational needs. At any point during their stay, youths can be transferred to a psychiatric hospital if needed. Otherwise they return home with a plan for outpatient mental health services, with aftercare services by the RISE program as appropriate. The length of stay may range from a few days to months. COMPASS is also operated by Seneca through a direct contract with VCBH: at this point only youths with Medi-Cal are eligible, but VCBH is exploring contracts with private insurance carriers as well.

The RISE program was developed as an innovative outreach engagement and referral team to serve Ventura County individuals of all ages who are having difficulty accessing mental health services. Referral sources include EDs, law enforcement, psychiatric hospitals, NAMI and other family/peer support groups, schools, and the CSU and COMPASS programs. Providers for the RISE program assess an individual's basic needs, provide connection to resources (eg, to food bank, bus tokens, shelter,

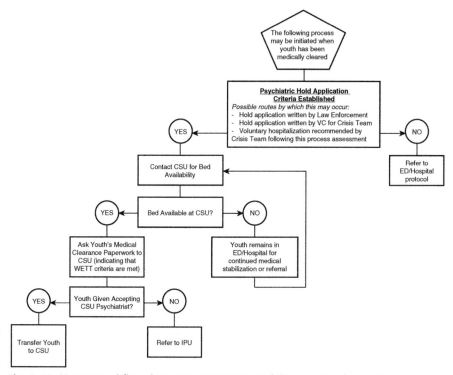

Fig. 4. ED CSU protocol flow chart. CSU, VCBH Crisis Stabilization Unit (psychiatric treatment for youth 6–17 years (regardless of insurance); ED, emergency department; IPU, inpatient psychiatric unit; VCBH, Ventura County Behavioral Health; WEFT, walk, eat, talk, toilet.

transportation), and refer to outpatient mental health services. Parent Partners from United Parents, a local peer support nonprofit agency contracted with VCBH, work closely with the RISE team to encourage increased caregiver involvement through the shared experience of raising a child with mental health challenges. RISE staff and Parent Partners can initiate contact with youths and families during hospitalization or in the CSU or COMPASS program. It is funded through a state crisis services grant awarded to VCBH as well as direct billing to MediCal.

Data

Between May 2016 and June 2017, the Mobile Crisis Team responded by phone or in person to 1503 calls; 33% of calls originated from local EDs, 24% from school, 16% from an outpatient treatment provider, 12% from a family member, and 12% from law enforcement (**Fig. 5**). Fifty-eight percent of the calls involved a youth already enrolled in services through VCBH.

In terms of insurance status, 66% had MediCal, 25% private insurance, and 9% were uninsured or unknown insurance status.

Eighty-four percent of the calls were due to concerns about self-harm and 13% percent for harm to others. The Mobile Crisis Team responded in person to 84% of the calls. Regarding crisis resolution, 52% of the calls were stabilized in the community, 24% were hospitalized involuntarily, 5% hospitalized voluntarily, and 16% were resolved by phone intervention (**Fig. 6**).

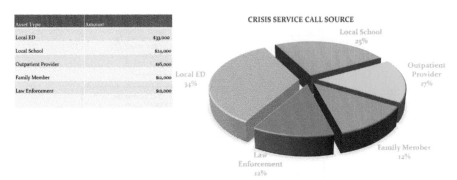

Asset Type	Amount
Local ED	$33,000
Local School	$24,000
Outpatient Provider	$16,000
Family Member	$12,000
Law Enforcement	$12,000

CRISIS SERVICE CALL SOURCE

Fig. 5. Crisis service: call source.

For the CSU, in 2016 to 2017, there were 241 admissions (47 of these readmissions). With regard to insurance status, 67% of youths had MediCal and 33% had private or no insurance. Girls accounted for 58% of the admissions, and 82% were aged 12 to 17 years. Half of the youths identified themselves as Latino. The most common primary admitting diagnoses were depressive disorder (61%), anxiety/stress related/adjustment disorder (21%), conduct disorder (4%), nonspecific mood disorder (4%), bipolar disorder (2%), and attention-deficit/hyperactivity disorder (2%). Approximately 56% were admitted on an involuntary hold. In terms of disposition, 62% were successfully diverted from an inpatient hospitalization.

For COMPASS, in the first 3 months, 4 youths were admitted; the initial was an especially aggressive child who required a high level of attention, preventing any other admissions for almost 2 months while awaiting placement in an out-of-state residential treatment center.

CONNECTICUT'S MOBILE CRISIS INTERVENTION SERVICE
Overview

Connecticut's Mobile Crisis Intervention Services (Mobile Crisis) is a core element of the state's children's behavioral health service array, funded and overseen by the

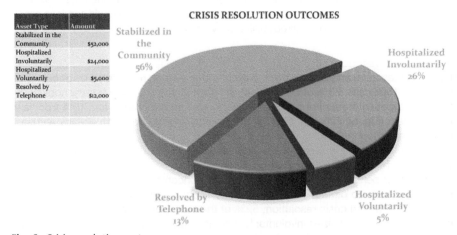

CRISIS RESOLUTION OUTCOMES

Asset Type	Amount
Stabilized in the Community	$52,000
Hospitalized Involuntarily	$24,000
Hospitalized Voluntarily	$5,000
Resolved by Telephone	$12,000

Fig. 6. Crisis resolution outcomes.

Connecticut Department of Children and Families (DCF). Connecticut DCF is one of the country's few consolidated children's agencies, with statutory responsibility for child protection, children's behavioral health, and substance abuse services and prevention. Connecticut's Mobile Crisis service embodies many of the best practices identified by SAMHSA, including 24/7 availability, rapid deployment to home or community locations, warm phone lines, crisis stabilization, crisis safety planning, short-term treatment, and linkage to ongoing care.[4]

A key feature of Connecticut's model is that the caller, not the call center intake specialists or responding providers, defines what constitutes a crisis. In many crisis response services, calls are triaged by varying criteria, often including a determination by the provider as to whether the call represents a true crisis. By allowing a crisis event to be defined by the caller, referrals are infrequently screened out, which helps to cilitate early identification and intervention and allows children and families broader access to the behavioral health system. To further support accessibility and convenience, Mobile Crisis is available free of charge to all children in the state younger than 18 years (or younger than 19 years if still enrolled in school) regardless of system involvement, insurance type, or ability to pay. Connecticut DCF provides sufficient grant funds to Mobile Crisis providers to ensure this level of accessibility, and providers supplement DCF grant funds with third-party reimbursement from Medicaid and commercial insurance.

The primary goals of Mobile Crisis are to keep children out of the ED, inpatient hospitals, and out-of-home placement, whenever community-based service delivery can be provided as a safe and effective alternative. Mobile Crisis service providers collaborate closely with families, community services and supports, schools, and EDs.

Program Details

Connecticut's Mobile Crisis system has 3 core components. The first is the provider network, which is organized around 6 primary contractors that collectively operate 14 sites, strategically located throughout the state to ensure full geographic coverage and the capacity for rapid response. Mobile crisis sites are generally located within large community mental health centers for children that operate a broad array of mental health and substance abuse services. Each of the 6 primary contractors employs a Mobile Crisis Director, site supervisors, and a sufficient number of master's level licensed (or license-eligible) clinicians to meet the demand at peak hours. In addition, each Mobile Crisis contract provides for dedicated psychiatric consultation with a board-certified child and adolescent psychiatrist. Following the initial response, clinicians can work with a family for up to 6 weeks, although the average service duration is 2 to 3 weeks. Core services include rapid mobile response, crisis stabilization, brief treatment, and referral and linkage to ongoing care.

The second component of the Mobile Crisis system is the statewide call center. Referrers can access Mobile Crisis by dialing 2-1-1 anywhere in the state. The statewide call center is open 24/7 and is operated by the United Way of Connecticut; it is staffed by trained intake clinicians. Hours of mobility are 6 AM to 10 PM on weekdays and 1 PM to 10 PM on weekends and holidays. For calls fielded during mobile hours, the 2-1-1-intake clinician collects basic information, including name, age, location, and the nature of the concern. Then the call is transferred to the appropriate mobile crisis provider for that child's location. For calls that arrive during nonmobile hours (4.5% of all calls), the caller speaks to the intake specialist, who then notifies the local provider for follow-up during mobile hours the following day.

The third component of Connecticut's Mobile Crisis system is the Performance Improvement Center (PIC). The PIC is housed at the Child Health and Development Institute of Connecticut and is responsible for data analysis, reporting, quality improvement activities, standardized practice development, and workforce development. The 2-1-1 and Mobile Crisis providers record information for every episode of care in DCF's Web-based data collection system; the PIC extracts those data for analysis of key indicators, including sociodemographic and clinical characteristics, performance measures, and outcomes. Key performance measures include benchmarks, such as episode volume, mobile response rates, and mobile response times. Mobile Crisis providers are required under contract with DCF to provide a mobile response to at least 90% of all calls and to arrive on site in 45 minutes or less for at least 80% of all mobile responses. Performance indicators and other data elements are reported on a monthly, quarterly, and annual basis for the statewide network, for each of the 6 contracted service areas and each of the14 provider sites. Data are shared openly and transparently with all providers and DCF and are made available to the public at www.empsct.org. Those data are used to inform the development of quarterly performance improvement plans.

Data

Since robust data collection on the service began in fiscal year 2010, Mobile Crisis has provided 81,400 episodes of care. In fiscal year 2017 alone, Mobile Crisis provided 13,461 episodes of care, a rate of 16.5 per 1000 children in the state and 31.65 per 1000 among children living in poverty (**Fig. 7**).

Approximately 40% of referrals to Mobile Crisis are from families and 35% are from schools; approximately 65% are enrolled in Medicaid and 30% are privately insured. Mobile Crisis serves a roughly equivalent number of boys and girls; the largest proportion of youths served are 13 to 15 years old (33.2%). Of the children for whom race was reported, most of the children served were white (62.0%), followed by black (23.0%) and other race (12.1%). Approximately 32% of youths served identified as Hispanic (any race). Importantly, the percentage of youths served by the Mobile Crisis who identify as black or Hispanic is higher than the percentage in the statewide population (46% of children served by Mobile Crisis are black or Hispanic compared with 34% of the statewide population composed of black and Hispanic youths), in contrast to many behavioral health programs that tend to underserve youths of color.[5–8] On key

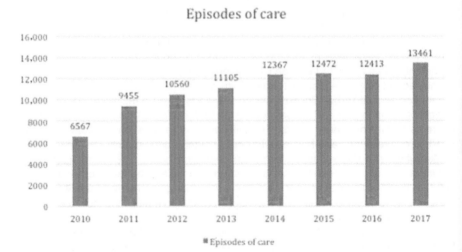

Fig. 7. Number of episodes of care by year.

performance indicators, all 6 service areas met or exceeded the benchmark that at least 90% of referrals will result in a mobile response (statewide average of 93%) as well as the benchmark that at least 80% of all mobile responses will occur in 45 minutes or less (statewide average of 88%, median response time of 27 minutes). With respect to the estimated cost savings of Mobile Crisis, in fiscal year 2017, 449 referrals were inpatient diversions. Of these referrals, 62% (278) were youths enrolled in Medicaid. These diversions resulted in an estimated saving of $2,945,966 in Medicaid costs.

SUMMARY/DISCUSSION

Recent data indicate that many children and families first seek mental health care in emergency settings; this can be associated with less favorable clinical outcomes and can be financially taxing.[1,9] Thus, communities can benefit from the development and expansion of a continuum of nonhospital youth psychiatric crisis care services to better meet their needs. As reviewed in this article, there are multiple types of crisis services, ranging from phone triage lines, to mobile crisis units, to brief stabilization and observation units for youths. By using a continuum of crisis services, communities can help divert youths away from EDs, provide the most appropriate level of evaluation and assessment, and refer and coordinate to longer-term outpatient services.

For communities hoping to expand community crisis services, collaborating with key local stakeholders, identifying funding sources, evaluating/leveraging existing services, and expanding staffing and training are important foundational tenants. Hospitals and communities can establish clear policies and practices to ensure early identification of youths who are appropriate for diversion from the ED and toward community-based alternatives, whenever these services can be provided as a safe and effective alternative. The community can also improve education around appropriate use of the ED, how to access community-based alternatives, and also to help communities formalize linkages between hospitals and community-based resources.

REFERENCES

1. Torio CM, Encinosa W, Berdahl T, et al. Annual report on health care for children and youth in the United States: national estimates of cost, utilization, and expenditures for children with mental health conditions. Acad Pediatr 2015;15(1):19–35.
2. Kim WJ, Bechtold D, Brooks BA, et al, American Academy of Child and Adolescent Psychiatry Task Force on Workforce Needs. Child and adolescent psychiatry workforce: a critical shortage and national challenge. Acad Psychiatry 2003;27:277–82.
3. Vanderploeg JJ, Lu JJ, Marshall JJ. Mobile crisis services for children and families: advancing a community-based model in Connecticut. Child Youth Serv Rev 2016; 71:103–9.
4. Substance Abuse and Mental Health Services Administration (SAMHSA) crisis services: effectiveness, cost-effectiveness, and funding strategies [Report No. (SMA)-14-4848]. Available at: http://store.samhsa.gov/product/Crisis-Services-Effectiveness-Cost-Effectiveness-and-Funding-Strategies/SMA14-4848. Accessed October 5, 2017.
5. U.S. Census Bureau (2016). Quick facts: Ventura County, California. Available at: https://www.census.gov/quickfacts/fact/table/venturacountycalifornia/PST045216. Accessed October 5, 2017.
6. Shannahan RS, Fields S. Services in support of community living for youth with serious behavioral health challenges: mobile crisis response and stabilization

services. Rockville (MD): Substance Abuse and Mental Health Services Administration; 2016.

7. Alegria M, Vallas M, Pumariega A. Racial and ethnic disparities in pediatric mental health child and adolescent psychiatric clinics. Child Adolesc Psychiatr Clin N Am 2010;19(4):759–74.

8. Marrast L, Himmelstein D, Woolhandler S. Racial and ethnic disparities in mental health care for children and young adults: a national study. Int J Health Serv 2016;46(4):810–24.

9. Gill PJ, Saunders NS, Gandhi S, et al. Emergency department as a first contact for mental health problems in children and youth. J Am Acad Child Adolesc Psychiatry 2017;56(6):475–82.e4.

Multidisciplinary Approach to Enhancing Safety and Care for Pediatric Behavioral Health Patients in Acute Medical Settings

Gary Lelonek, MD[a],*, Douglas Crook, BSN, RN[b], Maura Tully, MSEd, CCLS[c], Kristen Trufelli, LMHC[d], Lindsay Blitz, BSN, RN[e], Steven C. Rogers, MD, MS-CTR[f]

KEYWORDS

- Security • Behavioral health • Emergency • Child life • Multidisciplinary teams
- Agitation • Simulation • Behavioral response team

KEY POINTS

- Behavioral response teams support patients and the medical team by providing expert guidance and assistance in treatment planning and during behavioral crises.
- Security department training focusing on recognizing early signs of agitation and developmental aspects of communication enhances patient and staff safety.
- Child life specialists support patients during their crisis visit, enhances coping skills, and prepares patients and families for procedures and admission using developmentally appropriate therapeutic activities.
- Dialectical behavioral therapy training for emergency department staff helps staff better understand emotional dysregulation and how to coach and support patients during their crisis visit.
- Agitation management simulations increase staff and trainee comfort and preparedness to work with agitated patients.

[a] Cohen Children's Medical Center, Northwell Health, 270-05 76th Avenue, New Hyde Park, NY 11040, USA; [b] Behavioral Response Team, Boston Children's Hospital, 300 Longwood Avenue, Boston, MA 02115, USA; [c] Child Life Department, Cohen Children's Medical Center of New York, 269-01 76th Avenue, New Hyde Park, NY 11040, USA; [d] Behavioral Health Urgent Care Center, Cohen Children's Medical Center of New York, 269-01 76th Avenue, New Hyde Park, NY 11040, USA; [e] Emergency Department, Connecticut Children's Medical Center, 282 Washington Street, Hartford, CT 06106, USA; [f] Division of Emergency Medicine, Emergency Mental Health Services, Connecticut Children's Medical Center, 282 Washington Street, Hartford, CT 06106, USA
* Corresponding author.
E-mail address: glelonek1@northwell.edu

Child Adolesc Psychiatric Clin N Am 27 (2018) 491–500
https://doi.org/10.1016/j.chc.2018.03.004   childpsych.theclinics.com

INTRODUCTION

Pediatric patients in behavioral health crises account for 5% of all pediatric emergency department (ED) visits and have doubled in the last 15 years.[1-3] The most common psychiatric diagnoses seen in the emergency setting are oppositional defiant disorder, depressive disorder, attention-deficit hyperactivity disorder, nonsuicidal self-injury, and suicide attempts.[3] EDs and medical inpatient units are anxiety-provoking for children owing to unfamiliar and often overwhelming environmental stimuli, pain, and loss of control, which can potentially trigger behavioral outbursts.[4] Agitation is triggered by anxiety, mood disorders, delirium, suicidal threats, disruptive behaviors, and alcohol or drug withdrawal. There are 1.7 million ED visits for agitation involving all diagnoses annually.[5] Treating patients with agitation is challenging because it threatens the safety of staff and patients. Agitated patients account for significant staff injuries and disability. In a survey across 65 EDs, 25% of ED staff reported feeling safe at work, "sometimes," "rarely," or "never."[6] In addition, the 2010 Emergency Nurses Association study on violence in the workplace reported that more than half of emergency nurses had been verbally or physically threatened at work within the preceding 7 days.[7] When facing an agitated pediatric patient, medical care providers often interact with them as if they were adults. Pediatric patients process information differently from adults, which affects their behaviors, especially during emotionally charged interactions, leading to erratic responses at times. Deescalating agitated children necessitates a neurodevelopmentally sensitive approach that considers the child's abilities, the time they require to process information, their need to have instructions repeated in a developmentally appropriate manner, and understanding that they often benefit from explanations, alternatives, and consequences.[8]

Staff members in acute medical settings often have difficulties caring for patients with various behavioral health issues. It has been shown that patients with self-injurious behaviors and suicidality, as well as patients' substance abuse issues, pose the biggest challenge to emergency care providers.[9] Despite the increasing number of mental health ED visits and decades of recommendations to improve the education of pediatric and emergency medicine residents regarding mental health issues, about 65% of pediatricians surveyed by the American Academy of Pediatrics indicated that they lacked training in recognizing and treating mental health problems.[10] Also, in the American Board of Emergency Medicine board certification examination, 4% or less of the questions pertain to behavioral issues.[11] Staff working in acute medical settings may not have the skills needed to recognize warning signs of escalating behavior or to deescalate potentially unsafe behavior.[12]

Several strategies may improve the quality of behavioral health care in the acute medical setting. These can include staff education, utilization of various deescalation techniques, and ensuring availability of specialized resources. This article describes multidisciplinary initiatives from 3 academic centers, each developed to improve how agitation and behavioral health patients are managed in acute pediatric settings. Boston Children's Hospital (BCH) has implemented the Behavioral Response Team (BRT), which is a consultative rapid response and supportive resource consisting of registered nurses and a milieu counselor with experience managing acute psychiatric disorders and agitation. The team works closely with physicians, social workers, and security officers in the ongoing and crisis care of patients with behavioral health needs.[13,14] At the Connecticut Children's Hospital, security team training initiatives include management of agitation in children, which has yielded improved outcomes. Northwell Health's Cohen Children's Medical Center has 3 relevant programs. First, child life specialists enhance and support the care of pediatric patients presenting with behavioral health complaints. Next, the education program teaches multidisciplinary staff the principles of Dialectical Behavior Therapy (DBT), affecting regulation skills and how these may be used when working with youth in crisis in the ED. Finally, agitation management simulations (AMSs), developed to help increase staff and trainee comfort and preparedness to work with agitated patients, are discussed.[15,16] Together, these initiatives decrease agitation morbidity and effect change in the alliance built with these patients and their families, as well as increase staff and trainee comfort and preparedness to work with agitated patients.[15,16]

BEHAVIORAL RESPONSE TEAM: BOSTON CHILDREN'S HOSPITAL

Rapid response teams have been used in medicine for several years. These teams of experts respond to medical emergencies early on and aim to provide expertise and assistance to patients who are decompensating. The use of a behavioral emergency rapid response team has been an effective means of addressing behavioral emergencies early on, decreasing the use of restraint, lessening the incidence of workplace violence, and reducing calls to security. A behavioral emergency rapid response team can also improve staff confidence in identifying, managing, and deescalating agitation.[12–14] In response to the growing number of behavioral health patients being cared for in the medical setting, BCH created the BRT. On implementation, the team consisted of 1 mental health nurse who worked with the patients throughout the enterprise. A 24-hour on-call emergency response team that was available as needed for emergent behavioral crisis focused on deescalation and management. The BRT has since expanded to a team of 5 nurses and 1 milieu counselor. The team provides both proactive and crisis behavioral health support throughout the day and evening. The BRT operates independently but in close collaboration with all departments, including psychiatry, the medical teams, security, and child life.

The BRT sees a variety of patients with or without a comorbid medical diagnosis. Early assessment and proactive treatment planning have been the most helpful in minimizing behavioral emergencies and facilitating safe admissions. Gathering information and including the family's input about a patient's behavior, triggers, and coping mechanisms allows tailoring of treatment plans. Having as much information as possible before episodes of agitation is also helpful when attempting to deescalate a situation because it is often difficult to obtain useful information when a patient is already agitated. Understanding as much as possible regarding early signs of anxiety or agitation, specific triggers, and effective coping mechanisms are all necessary for promoting safe and strength-based care.[17] The team at BCH found that nurses may spend less time with the behavioral health patient when the patient exhibits good behavioral control; however, time invested to build rapport is valuable and yields improved outcomes.

The team's milieu counselor works in the BCH ED. The counselor collaborates with the ED nursing team, physicians, child life specialists, and emergency psychiatry service to support patients presenting to the ED in acute behavioral health crises. Support plans are created for patients who are challenged by the ED environment and are expected to be waiting in the ED for an extended period of time. The BRT milieu counselor provides ongoing support in addition to assistance with management during episodes of behavioral crisis. The team also provides treatment plans for patients before planned hospital admissions. The BRT is often consulted before surgeries, same day procedures, and other appointments to provide input about how to best support patients through these interventions. The BRT will meet with patients and families during preprocedure visits or will complete planning by telephone. A detailed plan is made and recommendations are communicated to the medical team before scheduled appointments. Treatment plans are tailored based on risk level and can range from a brief support plan to a more detailed plan, including behavioral interventions and medication recommendations. The plans often include special accommodations to minimize overstimulation, such as the team meeting the patient outside the hospital and accompanying them to their destination, avoiding the lobby, using halls that have limited traffic, and ensuring available rooms so that waiting rooms can be bypassed. Despite extensive proactive planning, an emergent response is still needed at times. The BRT is available to support the pediatric teams and their patients through periods of crisis. BCH uses a code (the Behavioral Rapid Response), activated via the emergency page system, to alert the BRT, the psychiatry team, and security of a behavioral emergency. The BRT responds and works closely with the clinical team to resolve the situation. Large numbers of people can be overwhelming for the patient and cause further behavioral escalation, so it is important to assess the number of people required to manage the situation. Additionally, overwhelmed patients may not hear and integrate information easily, so it is helpful to remind staff to use short and concrete language with the patient.[18] These 2 points are critical not only in managing the patient but also in supporting the staff, who may be unsure about how to best care for the patient and manage potentially unsafe behavior. Identifying a leader is an effective way to maintain control of a situation. The leader can delegate tasks to others (eg, obtaining orders, preparing medications, minimizing environmental stimulation) while he or she provides direct support to the patient and makes attempts at behavioral deescalation. The BRT will help lead the team or support the team member with the best rapport who may have already taken on this role.

Introducing the BRT has been helpful across the hospital in managing behavioral crises in the various medical settings and is perceived as a helpful resource by pediatric providers and families.

INNOVATION IN SECURITY CURRICULUM: CONNECTICUT CHILDREN'S MEDICAL CENTER

Over the past 5 years, the security department of Connecticut Children's Medical Center has innovated safety monitoring and interventions. A 5-member behavioral health ED security division was developed to address the hospital's increasing emergency department behavioral health population. The team was trained through observation and video surveillance to recognize early signs of agitation and to initiate verbal deescalation efforts. The security curriculum focuses on training officers to maintain patient safety through an empathetic attitude. Courses are titled "Safety Starts with Me" and "Start with Heart." The classes demonstrate therapeutic techniques such as rapport building and active listening. In addition, the staff receives certification in crisis prevention intervention training, which is known to emphasize increasing self and environmental awareness, and to focus on facilitating deescalation mediations rather than immediate physical actions.[12,19] Team members cultivate the ability to detect escalating behaviors and signs of increasing emotional distress. Officers can recognize the early signs of irritability and frustration, and can intervene before the situation escalates. They are trained to offer developmentally appropriate alternatives to relieve stress and diffuse the situation, including attending to the physical and emotional needs of the patient or using distraction techniques. Preemptive intervention has a greater rate of success in alleviating the patient's stress and decreases use of physical holds and restraints. However, instances occur in which the use of physical interventions is unavoidable. The goal in these situations is to ensure that they are implemented safely in alignment with hospital policies. The training program also focuses on teaching security officers to practice safe, age-appropriate means for restraining children and adolescents. The security department also has a joint education program with the local police department on how to cautiously and appropriately secure a patient attempting to cause harm to themselves and/or others. In addition to adhering to proper defense tactics, these joint trainings allow them to gain a foundational understanding of the factors involved in deescalation, including when and how to disengage and/or reengage with a patient. The security curriculum development and the team's continuous expansion (there are now 30 officers trained across multiple locations) and progress over the past 5 years exemplify their dedication to patient and staff safety. The education protocols and practical training on the use of restraints and deescalation, along with the collaboration with law enforcement, has decreased the use of restraints and staff injuries to a historical low and has increased the feeling of staff preparedness, comfort, and safety working with agitated patients at the institution.

INITIATIVES: COHEN CHILDREN'S MEDICAL CENTER
Child Life and Behavioral Health in the Emergency Department

The focus of child life specialists is to increase a pediatric patient's understanding of their hospital experience, as well as to support their adaptive coping skills. The 3 key elements of the preparation process are the dissemination of developmentally appropriate information, the encouragement of questions and emotional expression, and the formation of a trusting relationship with a health care professional.[20] Although these services are generally thought of as applicable to medical or surgical patients, they are increasingly applied to meet the needs of the behavioral health population. A concentrated effort has been put forth in the last 5 years by the child life team at Cohen Children's Medical Center to provide assessments for and interventions with behavioral health patients to help support this population during their crisis visit to the ED.

In the Northwell Health Pediatric ED, the child life specialists work in close collaboration with the behavioral health providers. When behavioral health patients require support through the various stages of their ED evaluation, the child life specialists are able to provide assistance. The assistance of a child life specialist may be needed during medical clearance or interventions, understanding the hospital process, preparation for procedures, procedural support during computed tomography scans and intravenous tube placements, preparation for hospital admissions (including psychiatric admissions using pictures of the unit and sharing schedules and programming), and general emotional support. Patients who present for anxiety, depression, and so forth are asked a series of open-ended questions, seeking information regarding what helps them to cope in general, in the hospital environment, or in general during times of stress. A coping plan is developed and implemented, giving these patients a sense of choice and control in a situation that often strips them of these feelings.

Child life specialists also provide services to patients who have autism or other developmental delays. An informal assessment is done to see how the patient best communicates, what his or her potential triggers are, whether or not there are any major safety concerns, and how the patient best copes in the hospital environment. Parents and/or caregivers are seen as excellent resources by the child life specialist in regard to both assessment and intervention with developmentally delayed patients.[21] Information is gleaned from conversations with parents about previous reactions to health care environments, as well as about what adjustments to the environment or to the approach of the staff could be made to reduce the patient's stress and/or facilitate cooperation during the visit. Information is also solicited in regard to what diversionary activities the patient best responds. The provision of such activities is meant to keep the patient calm and, therefore, more cooperative with examination and required medical intervention.[22]

Patients in the behavioral health section of the pediatric ED may be required to remain there for extensive amounts of time while waiting for placement in an inpatient setting when admission is necessary. These extensive wait times in an isolated setting are difficult for patients and may increase feelings of anxiety and agitation. Child life specialists provide patients with diversionary activities to help minimize stress and maximize adaptive coping in these circumstances.

Developed by the Association of Child Life Professionals, many of the 2017 Standards of Clinical Practice,[23] as they relate to child life services, are not only applicable but are beneficial to the behavioral health population. Psychological preparation for potentially stressful experiences, support during identified stress points, stress reduction techniques to facilitate adaptive coping, and normalization of the environment, as well as the orientation to the setting in which care will occur, are all a part of the standard of clinical practice for child life specialists. These standards, when used by the child life team in conjunction with the multidisciplinary staff who use various modalities of intervention in their respective scopes of practice, help to decrease the stress and anxiety associated with a behavioral health evaluation in the pediatric ED, and supports patients with developmental or psychological concerns who have come to be seen for medical issues.

Dialectical Behavior Therapy Skills in the Management of Behavioral Health Emergencies

DBT is a comprehensive, evidenced-based treatment originally developed for use with chronically suicidal individuals diagnosed with borderline personality disorder.[24] The standard model of DBT consists of 4 modes of treatment: individual and family psychotherapy, skills training, telephone coaching, and a consultation team. DBT skills training alone has since been studied and implemented in treatment with a broad range of diagnoses and shown to be a promising intervention for a variety of populations. DBT skills training has been shown effective with eating disorders, treatment-resistant depression, and a variety of other disorders.[25] Standard DBT skills training consists of 5 modules of skills for adolescents: mindfulness, distress tolerance, emotion regulation, interpersonal effectiveness, and middle path. Skills target 5 areas of dysregulation: emotional, behavioral, interpersonal, self, and cognitive. The ED is an ideal setting for the use of DBT because of the focus on crisis suicidal behaviors. Patients in the ED are in heightened attentional and emotional states, which more readily lend themselves to the learning and synthesis of new skills.[26]

To manage behavioral dysregulation, Cohen Children's Medical Center behavioral health staff members are being taught DBT skills, distress tolerance, and milieu coaching. Adopted from the inpatient adolescent unit staff training materials, behavioral health staff members, including psychiatrists, nurses, residents, fellows, social workers, child life staff, and nurse practitioners, are oriented in 1-hour to 2-hour sessions in distress tolerance skills (TIPP [Temperature, Intense exercise, Paced breathing, Paired Muscle relaxation], self soothe, and ACCEPTS distracting skills [Activities, Contributing, Comparisons, opposite Emotions, Pushing away, Thoughts, Sensations] with Wise Mind) and skills coaching. Staff members are provided skills worksheets from the *DBT Skills Manual for Adolescents*[25] and coping materials to use with patients. Distress tolerance skills target behavioral dysregulation that results in suicide attempts or threats, nonsuicidal self-injury, aggression, and impulsive behaviors. Distress tolerance skills are acceptance-based skills that teach individuals to identify a crisis or stressful situation and tolerate strong negative emotions while avoiding dysfunctional behaviors that could make a situation worse.[27] The goal of these skills is to aid the patient in tolerating the distress without it leading to behavioral dysregulation (self-injury, suicide attempt, aggression). In standard DBT practice, skills training is conducted in a group therapy format. In Cohen Children's Medical Center's application, skills are used during individual interactions with patients in the ED, such as during assessment interviews, extended waiting times, safety planning, and discharge discussions. Coping kits have been created to provide patients with tools (eg, fidget toys, soft animals, stress balls, coloring books) for distraction, stress release, and self-soothing. Educating the staff regarding these principles has been helpful in promoting a culture change but the impact on patient satisfaction and safety measures is yet to be studied.

Agitation Management Simulations

Agitation is a psychiatric emergency. As with most medical emergencies, early recognition of the developing situation and calm collaboration of competent team members is of outmost importance in successful management of the emergency. When humans perceive threat, the sympathetic nervous system is activated, initiating a flight-or-fight response for both the patient and the providers. Managing agitation requires the acquisition of deescalation skills and self-regulation. Simulations are used in military training, aviation, and in medicine to prepare trainees and professionals. Preparing for situations with agitated patients requires training in scenarios that mimic the intensity of interactions with agitated patients.[15,16] AMSs were developed to increase the pediatric and behavioral health teams' (staff and trainees) comfort and preparedness to work with agitated patients, with the ultimate goal of decreasing agitation morbidity and effecting change in the alliances built.

An important consideration when working with patients who present with behavioral health emergencies is that up to 90% of them have experienced trauma; therefore, a trauma-informed approach is crucial in the management to decrease the detrimental effects on the patients and increase awareness of triggers.[28] To achieve this, the staff must collaborate with the agitated patient to help identify coping skills and triggers, and inquire about what is bothering them. Verbal deescalation skills need to be taught and reinforced annually.[18,29] These codes reinforce the concept that deescalation occurs in a repetitive cycle of listening, validating, and shaping. The agitation codes allow the staff the flexibility to address the needs of the patient while providing a clear algorithm that enhances patient and staff safety. The focuses of the simulation are maintaining clear and calm communication with the patient and hospital staff, decreasing agitation, increasing safety, and empathizing with the patient.[28]

Psychiatry and nursing staff designed 2 clinical scenarios. One scenario allows for successful verbal deescalation and the second scenario ends with the use of restraints. The actors in the scenarios are the ED clinical staff with experience working with agitated patients. The first scenario begins with a nurse alerting the doctor that a patient is agitated. The staff, led by a team leader, addresses environmental safety while simultaneously engaging the patient by assessing his or her needs. Environmental safety includes removing potentially dangerous items from the room, alerting support staff to help, and removing any triggers. Based on the verbal and nonverbal cues of the patient, the team leader determines whether the deescalation practices are stabilizing the patient's behavior. If the patient remains agitated but in behavioral control, the patient is offered symptom-focused treatment with medications based on the BETA (Best practices in Evaluation and Treatment of Agitation) recommendations.[30] In the second scenario the patient remains agitated and exhibits further verbal or behavioral escalation, and the leader communicates with the team about proceeding to the use of restraints. The team leader assigns each team member a specific role and designates a trigger phrase to start the restraint.

After each scenario, the actors and the AMS staff debrief with the team, modeling this crucial element of agitation management incidents. They give feedback about the effectiveness of the deescalation techniques and restraint implementation. The AMSs run twice every 10 weeks as new child psychiatry trainees circulate through the ED. They are joined by security personnel, pediatric emergency medicine doctors and nurses, support staff, and pediatric inpatient staff and trainees. In addition to the AMSs, the trainees participate in didactic learning sessions regarding agitation management, psychopharmacology, and other skills. This repeating cycle allows new trainees and regular staff to practice deescalation skills, as well as prepare for use of medication and restraints together.

SUMMARY

Emergency nurses and nonpsychiatric physicians commonly perceive themselves as lacking the knowledge, skills, and expertise to provide appropriate care and treatment to psychiatric emergency pediatric patients.[31–34] Lack of educational preparation in the care of psychiatric patients is frequently cited as an important contributing factor. The perspectives and initiatives described by these multidisciplinary teams may form a Managing Mental Health Crises Curriculum for psychiatry residency, security, nursing, and mental health professionals to gain competence in working with pediatric behavioral health patients.

REFERENCES

1. Carubia B, Becker A, Levine BH. Child psychiatric emergencies: updates on trends, clinical care, and practice challenges. Curr Psychiatry Rep 2016;18:41.
2. Grupp-Phelan J, Harman JS, Kelleher KJ. Trends in mental health and chronic condition visits by children presenting for care at U.S. emergency departments. Public Health Rep 2007;122(1):55–61.
3. Mahajan P, Alpern ER, Grupp-Phelan J, et al. Epidemiology of psychiatric-related visits to emergent departments in a multicenter collaborative research pediatric network. Pediatr Emerg Care 2009;25(11):715–20.
4. Nager AL, Mahrer NE, Gold JI. State trait anxiety in the emergency department: an analysis of anticipatory and life stressors. Pediatr Emerg Care 2010;26:897–901.
5. Allen MH, Currier GW, Carpenter D, et al. Expert consensus panel for behavioral emergencies 2005. J Psychiatr Pract 2005;11(Suppl 1):5–108 [quiz: 110–2].
6. Kansagra SM, Rao SR, Sullivan AF, et al. A survey of workplace violence across 65 U.S. emergency departments. Acad Emerg Med 2008;15:1268–74.
7. Emergency Nurses Association Institute for Emergency Nursing Research. Emergency department violence surveillance study. Available at: http://www.ena.org/IENR/Documents/ENAEVSSReportAugust2010.pdf. Accessed February 24, 2011.
8. Bostic JQ, Thurau L, Potter M, et al. Policing the teen brain. J Am Acad Child Adolesc Psychiatry 2014;53(2):127–9.
9. Emergency Nurses Association. White paper on care of the psychiatric patient in the emergency department. Available at: https://www.ena.org/practice-research/research/Documents/WhitePaperCareofPsych.pdf. Accessed December 12, 2015.

10. McMillan JA, Land M, Leslie LK. Pediatric residency education and the behavioral and mental health crisis: a call to action pediatrics. Pediatrics 2017;139(1) [pi:e20162141].

11. Zun L. Care of psychiatric patients: the challenge to emergency physicians. West J Emerg Med 2016;17(2):173–6.

12. Zicko JM, Schroeder RA, Byers WS, et al. Behavioral emergency response team: implementation improves patient safety, staff safety, and staff collaboration. Worldviews Evid Based Nurs 2017;14(5):377–84.

13. Loucks J, Rutledge DN, Hatch B, et al. Rapid response team for behavioral emergencies. J Am Psychiatr Nurses Assoc 2010;16(2):93–100.

14. Pestka EL, Hatteberg DA, Larson LA, et al. Enhancing safety in behavioral emergency situations. Medsurg Nurs 2012;21(6):335–41. Available at: http://www.medsurgnursing.net.

15. Wong AH, Wing L, Weiss B, et al. Coordinating a team response to behavioral emergencies in the emergency department: a simulation-enhanced interprofessional curriculum. West J Emerg Med 2015;16(6):859–65.

16. Healea B. Off the verge: teaching De-escalation through simulation; 2017. Available at: Honors Projects Overview. 129. https://digitalcommons.ric.edu/honors_projects/129. Accessed April 18, 2018.

17. LeBel J. Child and adolescent inpatient restraint reduction: a state initiative to promote strength-based care. J Am Acad Child Adolesc Psychiatry 2004;43(1):37–45.

18. Richmond JS, Berlin JS, Fishkind AB, et al. Verbal De-escalation of the agitated patient: consensus statement of the American Association for Emergency Psychiatry Project BETA De-escalation workgroup. West J Emerg Med 2012;13(1):17–25.

19. Gillam SW. Nonviolent crisis intervention training and the incidence of violent events in a large hospital emergency department: an observational quality improvement study. Adv Emerg Nurs J 2014;36:177–88.

20. AAP News and Journals Gateway, 2017. Available at: www.childlife.org. Accessed January 3, 2018.

21. Horowitz L, Kassam-Adams N, Bergstein J. Mental health aspects of emergency medical services for children: summary of a consensus conference. J Pediatr Psychol 2001;26(8):491–502.

22. Chun TH, Katz ER, Duffy SJ, et al. Challenges of managing pediatric mental health crises in the emergency department. Child Adolesc Psychiatr Clin N Am 2015;24(1):21–40.

23. Standards of Clinical Practice, Association of Child Life Professionals. 2017.

24. Linehan MM. DBT® skills training manual. 2nd edition. New York: Guilford Press; 2015.

25. Rathus JH, Miller AL. DBT® skills manual for adolescents. New York: Guilford Press; 2015.

26. Sneed JR, Balestri M, Belfi BJ. The use of dialectical behavior therapy strategies in the psychiatric emergency room. Psychother Theor Res Pract Train 2003;40(4): 265–77.

27. Valentine SE, Bankoff SM, Poulin RM, et al. The use of dialectical behavior therapy skills training as stand-alone treatment: a systematic review of the treatment outcome literature. J Clin Psychol 2015;71(1):1–20.

28. Gallo K, Smith L. Building a culture of patient safety through simulation; an interprofessional learning model. Springer Publishing Company; 2014.

29. Allen M, Forster P, Zealberg J, et al. Report and recommendations regarding psychiatric emergency and crisis services: a review and model program descriptions. American Psychiatric Association Task Force on Psychiatric Emergency

Services Web site. Available at: http://www.emergencypsychiatry.org/data/tfr200201.pdf. Accessed June 13, 2011.

30. Wilson MP, Pepper D, Currier GW, et al. The psychopharmacology of agitation: consensus statement of the American Association for Emergency Psychiatry Project BETA psychopharmacology workgroup. West J Emerg Med 2012;13(1):26–34.

31. Clarke DE, Hughes L, Brown AM, et al. Psychiatric emergency nurses in the emergency department: the success of the Winnipeg, Canada, experience. J Emerg Nurs 2005;31(4):351–6.

32. Gordon JT. Emergency department junior medical staff's knowledge, skills and confidence with psychiatric patients: a survey. The Psychiatrist 2012;36(5):186–8.

33. Kerrison SA, Chapman R. What general emergency nurses want to know about mental health patients presenting to their emergency department. Accid Emerg Nurs 2007;15(1):48–55.

34. Wand T, Happell B. The mental health nurse: contributing to improved outcomes for patients in the emergency department. Accid Emerg Nurs 2001;9(3):166–76.

Training, Education, and Curriculum Development for the Pediatric Psychiatry Emergency Service

Amy Egolf, MD[a], Pamela Hoffman, MD[b],
Megan M. Mroczkowski, MD[c], Laura M. Prager, MD[d],
John W. Tyson Jr, MD[e], Kathleen Donise, MD[f],*

KEYWORDS

- Curriculum • Training and education • Emergency pediatric psychiatry
- Child psychiatry

KEY POINTS

- There is no standard care delivery model for pediatric psychiatric emergencies.
- With minimal directives, training programs lack guidance on developing optimal curricula for this setting.
- A model curriculum for child and adolescent psychiatry trainees must assess baseline knowledge, teach core subject content, encourage development of essential skills, and supervise learners.
- Future directions include further study in current pediatric emergency psychiatry education as well as expanding the scope and reach of curricula to different learners and delivery models.

Disclosure Statement: The authors report no relationship with a commercial company that has a direct financial interest in subject matter or materials discussed in article or with a company making a competing product.

[a] Department of Psychiatry and Human Behavior, Warren Alpert Medical School at Brown University, 593 Eddy Street, Providence, RI 02903, USA; [b] Hasbro Psychiatric Emergency Services, Department of Psychiatry and Human Behavior, Warren Alpert Medical School at Brown University, 593 Eddy Street, Main 038, Providence, RI 02903, USA; [c] Pediatric Psychiatry Emergency Service, Morgan Stanley Children's Hospital, New York Presbyterian Hospital, Columbia University Medical Center, 3959 Broadway CHONY 6 North, New York, NY 10032, USA; [d] Child Psychiatry Emergency Service, Transitional Age Youth Clinic, Harvard Medical School, Massachusetts General Hospital, 55 Fruit Street, Yawkey 6900, Boston, MA 02114, USA; [e] Division of Child and Adolescent Psychiatry, Massachusetts General Hospital, 55 Fruit Street, YAW6A, Boston, MA 02114, USA; [f] Lifespan Pediatric Behavioral Health Emergency Services, Department of Psychiatry and Human Behavior, Warren Alpert Medical School at Brown University, Rhode Island Hospital, Main Building, Room #038, 593 Eddy Street, Providence, RI 02903, USA
* Corresponding author.
E-mail address: kdonise@lifespan.org

Child Adolesc Psychiatric Clin N Am 27 (2018) 501–509
https://doi.org/10.1016/j.chc.2018.02.006
1056-4993/18/© 2018 Elsevier Inc. All rights reserved.

BACKGROUND AND RELEVANCE

Emergency child psychiatry is growing in importance and relevance. There is increased use of the emergency department (ED), both as a site for child and adolescent crisis evaluation and also as a front door to mental health services.[1,2] Training in this area is relevant for all mental health professionals who may treat children. Child and adolescent psychiatrists will especially benefit from this education, as even those who do not work primarily in the ED will use learned crisis skills while taking calls, working within a group, or practicing individually.

There are multiple models for service delivery of emergency psychiatric care. These models include mobile crisis services in the community, freestanding crisis centers, psychiatric consultation to the emergency department, separate locked psychiatric areas within the ED, and specialized comprehensive psychiatric emergency programs.[3] Additionally, children and adolescents receive evaluations in different ways. Some programs use social workers to triage and assess patients and determine appropriate disposition, whereas others consult psychiatry for each patient with a behavioral health chief complaint. Within each of these settings, there may be various types of front-line care providers at distinct levels of training, including but not limited to: social workers, licensed mental health workers, advanced practice nurses (APRNs), psychology trainees, medical students, adult psychiatry residents, residents from alternate disciplines, child psychiatry fellows, and attending child and/or adult psychiatrists. These front-line providers may report to various people in different specialties, such as ED physicians, senior-level child and adolescent psychiatry trainees, and attending psychiatrists.

INTRODUCTION TO CURRICULUM DEVELOPMENT IN EMERGENCY PSYCHIATRY

Given there is no one standard delivery model for psychiatric emergencies, many different education and curriculum models have been developed to address the individual system needs of each training program. Several emergency psychiatry services have created boot camp curricula targeting first-year child psychiatry fellows in the first few months of training. This curriculum typically contains information about the highest yield topics, such as managing agitation, assessing suicide and homicide risk, and identifying legal and other issues within the specific system of care. Alternatively, other services have created educational opportunities within the rotation itself. These opportunities typically include a detailed approach to pertinent topics, such as communication and triage, risk assessment, workup for first-break psychosis, legal issues specific to the ED, and child protective laws. Many programs use both models.

Educators are responsible for producing core learning outcomes for their medical curricula.[4] The Accreditation Council for Graduate Medical Education (ACGME) has published vague guidelines on the necessary elements of education in emergency child psychiatry: "Fellows must have an organized educational clinical experience in...initial management of psychiatric emergencies in children and adolescents."[5] ACGME expects trainees to demonstrate proficiency in 6 core competency areas of medical knowledge, patient care, practice-based learning and improvement, interpersonal and communication skills, professionalism, and systems-based practice. Beyond this, there are no formal curricular objectives for emergency child psychiatric care.

With minimal directives, programs lack guidance on developing optimal curricula for this setting. There is some guidance by way of general emergency psychiatry training curricula.[6–9] However, nothing to date has specifically addressed pediatric emergency psychiatry. Therefore, this group designed an informal survey distributed to American

Academy of Child and Adolescent Psychiatry emergency psychiatry subject matter experts to inquire about past and current educational experiences. All 23 respondents observed children in psychiatric emergencies in some capacity during fellowship. Fewer people (65%) recall having a formal child psychiatry ED rotation with dedicated staff teaching simultaneously. The results show that respondents also cared for children with psychiatric emergencies in other venues: 39% as part of an adult psychiatry ED rotation and 52% while on call and participating in other rotations. Although these results may be clouded in recall bias, they nonetheless guide recommendations. It is necessary to consider both general training models as well as prior educational experiences to formalize key elements in a curriculum for emergency child and adolescent psychiatry.

FRAMEWORK PROPOSAL

The authors propose that a curriculum in emergency psychiatry follow a specific framework to evaluate, educate, and assess learners. Based on results of the survey it is clear that there are a myriad of teaching approaches. Although many programs could not identify a structured curriculum, consistent themes emerged. Programs frequently identified the need for assessing baseline knowledge, teaching core subject content, developing essential skills, and supervising learners. These topics are in line with the 5 key curricular elements proposed by Bordage and Harris[10] that include competencies to be acquired, learners, assessment, conditions for learning, and the sociopolitical-cultural context in which learning occurs. All of these should be considered to create an effective model curriculum.

Baseline Assessment

The first step in developing a curriculum is to understand the individual learner's prior experience and knowledge to effectively tailor the current education. Learners may include junior and senior child psychiatry fellows, adult psychiatry residents, trainees from alternate specialties, and medical students. Within a single level of training, such as junior child psychiatry fellows, trainees come to a program with great variability in prior experience and knowledge. Even learners who evaluated children in an emergency setting may or may not have received formal teaching. Residencies provide different exposure to child emergency psychiatry. As evidence of this, among survey participants, one-third report having no formal rotation in child emergency psychiatry.

A baseline assessment should evaluate a learner's knowledge, skills, and attitudes, predicated on the training milestones. To focus a trainee's education efficiently, it is important to establish his or her understanding of child emergency psychiatry. Skills related to communication while working within a multidisciplinary team are also necessary to determine. Finally, assessing a trainee's attitude toward the field will provide a foundation to encourage sensitivity and professionalism. Such baseline assessment may be conducted via direct conversation with the trainee about prior experience, review of feedback about the trainee from other rotations, or a structured knowledge evaluation.

Orientation

Trainees need a general orientation to go over rules and expectations related to treating children and adolescents in crisis. Trainees must understand from the onset that unless the minor child is in acute danger, no decisions regarding psychopharmacologic treatment or plans regarding disposition can be made without the involvement of the legal guardian. A program must also familiarize trainees with local regulations, laws, and resources to guide education of relevant subject matter. Examples of regulations that may differ by state include requirements for consent and assent for voluntary hospitalization, involuntary commitment, confidentiality of children and adolescents, emancipation of minors, and mandated reporting of abuse. To effectively function, education in these local regulations is critical for the trainee, who may have had previous training elsewhere. Also, levels of care and local resources may be fewer or unavailable depending on the region and may affect patient management and disposition.

Core Subject Matter

Once a baseline assessment has been conducted and orientation completed, the authors propose a model curriculum contain specific core subject matter. A group of experts in pediatric emergency psychiatry compiled a list of core subject material, included in the survey. Despite the numerous ways in which material is delivered, a significant cohort of respondents deemed particular topics as critical; all agree risk assessment is necessary. For each topic offered in the survey, at least one-third agreed it was important. **Box 1** contains this list of core subject material.

Selected topics deserve further discussion. To start, though universally accepted, risk assessment is often reduced to suicidality. However, risk should address both harm to others and to self, accounting for patients' current environment. Patients who disclose unsafe behaviors or urges, such as engaging in self-harm or voicing homicidal ideation with a plan, may require environmental interventions. Until further evaluated, they need to be placed in a safe setting or assigned someone who can provide ongoing observation (eg, constant observation status with a sitter or 1:1 staff).

Management of agitation should always address behavioral and psychopharmacologic interventions. Education should also emphasize minimizing restraint and seclusion. Some pediatric patients who present to the ED with psychiatric crises may calm down quite quickly with simple interventions like attention, food, decreased stimulation, or containment. Alternatively, the same approach may cause other patients to become increasingly behaviorally dysregulated. Therefore, frequent assessments

---

Box 1
Core topics in pediatric emergency psychiatry

- Risk assessment
- Agitation
- Delirium
- Substance use
- Legal status
- Communication with ED staff
- Use of the medical record
- Abuse/neglect
- Psychopharmacology
- Medical workup of psychosis
- Management of acute psychiatric emergencies (eg, neuroleptic malignant syndrome, catatonia, serotonin syndrome)

over time can be helpful to determine the interventions that improve the patients' ability to settle down and which interventions trigger escalation.

Special populations seen in the ED deserve individualized attention in regard to multiple aspects of management (**Box 2**). For example, patients with autism spectrum diagnoses may be unable to tell the evaluator what is wrong; many will have difficulty with any transition, such as change of personnel or venue. These situations will require consideration and management in the ED setting.

Another important special population to consider in the ED includes children boarded awaiting psychiatric admission. In addition to the increasing number of children and adolescents presenting to EDs for emergency psychiatric evaluations, there is also a trend of increased boarding of these patients within the ED.[11,12] This trend may be due to the shortage of inpatient bed availability as well as the limited community resources that specialize in pediatric psychiatry. Hospitals manage pediatric psychiatric boarders differently, with some systems holding these children in the ED for days and sometimes weeks. Other hospital systems admit children to medical beds to await an available inpatient psychiatric bed; when such a team exists, these patients are managed by a pediatric psychiatric consult liaison service. Even for systems that generally admit patients to board, there are times when there are no boarding beds available, and so all systems may require management of these patients in the ED.

This circumstance shifts the ED role from short-term management with very brief interventions to one in which active management of these children requires multiple follow-up evaluations. As care transitions away from singular assessments, ongoing interventions are used so that children receive treatment while waiting. Frequent reassessments are critical, as an acute crisis may resolve while children wait in the ED. This passage of time also allows for medication adjustments, psychoeducation, and support for patients and families as well as respite for families. Trainees may not have previously encountered a situation requiring the utilization of inpatient skills while functioning within a busy and chaotic ED setting.

Lastly, many trainees may not have encountered children with significant trauma. Therefore, learning about trauma-informed care of children is also new. Trainees must appreciate the importance of screening for child abuse (physical, verbal, emotional, and sexual abuse and neglect), domestic violence, intimate partner violence, and peer violence. Once children have been screened in a thoughtful and

---

Box 2
Special populations in pediatric emergency psychiatry

- Patients with a diagnosis of autism spectrum disorder
- Younger patients (<5 years of age)
- Pregnant adolescents
- Medically compromised youths
- Patients with co-occurring psychiatric and substance issues (dual diagnosis patients)
- LGBTQ youths
- Boarders
- Children with history of trauma

Abbreviation: LGBTQ, lesbian, gay, bisexual, transgender, queer, and questioning.

sensitive manner, trainees need to understand reporting procedures for traumas disclosed to them by patients and families. All of this information is necessary to evaluate the patients and families in crisis.

Core Skill Set

Given the complexity and variety of cases seen in an ED, it is necessary for trainees to learn to triage, evaluate, and provide appropriate disposition planning for these patients and families in crisis. The first step in any evaluation is gathering basic information, including who is accompanying the patients, from where patients present, and who has legal decision-making rights. After obtaining this triage information, trainees must be able to perform an initial safety assessment, which will guide immediate decisions related to treatment and monitoring.

Completing an evaluation in the ED is based on consolidating various sources of information and, therefore, requires specific training. Few pediatric patients who present to the ED can provide a complete history. Therefore, collateral sources of information are crucial. These sources may include school counselors or teachers, mental health outpatient providers, pediatricians, and state agencies, such as child protective services, the department of mental health, or services related to developmental disabilities.

Trainees in a supervisory role may not see patients first hand and are instead presented information by an evaluator who lacks formal training to assess children for mental health problems. Therefore, trainees must be able to guide the evaluator through this process and then work with that provider to interpret the information to reach an appropriate and safe disposition.

In the ED, case formulation may reflect a working diagnosis rather than a conclusive one, as the evaluation is done in cross-section. Although trainees do not see patients longitudinally, they see patients at a critical time. Trainees must be willing to generate a broad differential diagnosis for a particular presentation, as the diagnostic formulation may change over time. For example, a presenting symptom of psychosis may indicate a primary psychotic, trauma-related, mood, or substance use disorder, which may not be immediately distinguishable. A biopsychosocial formulation provides a useful framework for understanding the current presentation and guides trainees in making more accurate and helpful recommendations for treatment and psychoeducation for families. Trainees must be skilled at pulling together multiple pieces of information, including the full history, collateral information, psychiatric review of systems, and mental status examination, to formulate the case and determine an appropriate disposition. Knowledge of the available resources within a particular area is vital to disposition planning. Systems of care for children in need of psychiatric services vary tremendously from city to city and state to state. Access to inpatient services, residential treatment, partial hospitalization, outpatient crisis supports, wraparound community services, and urgent clinic referrals are options considered in many cases, but their specific availability may determine what is ultimately recommended. The ability of families to access care is also variable and will affect treatment options. For example, if a parent or guardian does not have the means to transport the child to a specific program, the team must formulate an alternate disposition. Trainees also need to be able to communicate these recommendations to the appropriate parties, including patients, families, providers, schools, and state agencies.

All of this information is ultimately documented in the patients' health record. Review of documentation standards to support medicolegal decision-making is critical and can be site specific. A completed evaluation must be organized and coherent, as it will guide other clinicians in the ED, serve as a template for clinician communication, and assist future treatment providers. It must accurately reflect the formulation and disposition, including a clear rationale for the plan of care, a risk assessment, and referral options for admission (voluntary or involuntary) or discharge. Recommendations for medications or other management strategies for these patients while they remain in the ED must also be documented.

Rarely, trainees work in an independent pediatric psychiatry ED. More often, trainees work as consultants to other departments. This work requires the ability to communicate effectively with others who lack formal expertise in child psychiatry. As a critical part of the medical team, trainees are in a unique position to help distinguish a psychiatric presentation of a medical issue and prevent a premature psychiatric diagnosis. Trainees may also work within a multidisciplinary team. In this role they may lead the team, help consolidate medical information, make medication recommendations, or supervise other trainees.

Together, these skills help trainees in gathering, consolidating, disseminating, and documenting information obtained through assessment. All of these skills are essential to making an informed assessment and treatment plan for the child who presents to an ED with an acute psychiatric crisis (**Box 3**).

Supervision: Support, Feedback, and Evaluation

Providing support to trainees who see patients in the ED, as well as opportunities for feedback and evaluation, fosters an environment for learning. Support may include group supervision or a team rounds approach, whereby important or difficult cases can be discussed.[13] In other situations, individual supervision may be feasible. In either model, providing a safe space to discuss emotionally challenging cases, particularly those involving abuse and neglect, is essential for the continued growth and well-being of trainees. Ongoing support also helps trainees manage issues of burnout, which may be precipitated by high patient volume and severity; isolating, nontraditional work hours; and vicarious traumatization. Although essential to subject matter experts, survey respondents typically report that while they directly observe trainees (91%), less than half (45%) engage them in additional supervision sessions outside of clinical care.

Box 3
Core skill set components in pediatric emergency psychiatry

- Triage
  - Gather basic demographic information
  - Perform an initial safety assessment

- Evaluation
  - Obtain collateral information
  - Consult with other evaluators
  - Formulate case using a biopsychosocial model
  - Generate differential diagnosis

- Disposition planning
  - Understand local services
  - Understand family capability to access care
  - Communicate recommendations to family, providers, and school

- Document assessment
  - Compose risk formulation
  - Justify reason for level of care

In addition to support, supervision in various forms serves as an opportunity for feedback. Supervision within and outside of direct clinical care are two different yet equally important paradigms, which offer the opportunity for appropriate, relevant, and prompt feedback. For child psychiatry fellows, who are required by ACGME to perform clinical skills evaluations, the ED provides a rich environment to practice interviewing and examination skills. In some ED delivery models, a graduated experience of supervision allows trainees to develop their own teaching and supervisory skills. For example, a medical student sees a patient and discusses it with a resident, who then presents to an attending psychiatrist. This model allows for multiple opportunities for clinical and professional skills growth as well as formative feedback.

Last, summative assessment and reciprocal evaluations between trainees, supervisors, and the specific health system create opportunities for individual, program, and system-wide growth. This assessment can be solicited directly in the context of supervision or via survey (with the option for anonymity). These evaluations should be completed at distinct time periods, such as the beginning, midpoint, and end of a rotation. Appropriate supervision, timely feedback, and constructive evaluations foster a professional attitude and encourage effective and compassionate care.

FUTURE DIRECTIONS

This article is meant to provide guidance in designing a curriculum for trainees, based on limited existing publications and an informal survey to subject matter experts in pediatric emergency psychiatry. Although this is a starting point for these recommendations, more formal inquiry is necessary for guiding future directions in training and education. Additional research avenues could expound on current guidelines tailored to adult emergency psychiatry.

Another future opportunity includes expanding the delivery of this educational curriculum. Potential delivery models may vary between structured trainings to more technology-based training, which may include simulations, such as practice treating patients with an acute behavioral disturbance, web-based modules, and trainings via videoconferencing.[14]

The current scope herein has been limited to trainees. However, treatment teams are often multidisciplinary. Psychiatric ED teams may include social workers, licensed mental health clinicians, and APRNs. Curricula designed to educate other providers working in the ED are also essential. Given the dire shortage of child and adolescent psychiatrists, it is imperative to train other providers who evaluate children in crisis, such as pediatricians and family physicians. Future educational initiatives should be considered to target the specific clinical practice of these providers in the care of our patients.

REFERENCES

1. Pittsenbarger ZE, Mannix R. Trends in pediatric visits to the emergency department for psychiatric illnesses. Acad Emerg Med 2014;21(1):25–30.
2. Gill PJ, Saunders N, Gandhi S, et al. Emergency department as a first contact for mental health problems in children and youth. J Am Acad Child Adolesc Psychiatry 2017;56(6):475–82, e474.
3. Vanderploeg JJ, Lu JJ, Marshall TM, et al. Mobile crisis services for children and families: advancing a community-based model in Connecticut. Child Youth Serv Rev 2016;71:103–9.
4. Rees CE. The problem with outcomes-based curricula in medical education: insights from educational theory. Med Educ 2004;38(6):593–8.

5. ACGME. ACGME program requirements for graduate medical education in child and adolescent psychiatry. [PDF]. 2007; ACGME program requirements for graduate medical education in child and adolescent psychiatry. Available at: https://www.acgme.org/Portals/0/PFAssets/ProgramRequirements/405_child_and_adolescent_psych_2017-07-01.pdf. Accessed September 14, 2017.
6. Brasch J, Glick RL, Cobb TG, et al. Residency training in emergency psychiatry: a model curriculum developed by the education committee of the American Association for Emergency Psychiatry. Acad Psychiatry 2004;28(2):95–103.
7. Brasch JS, Ferencz JC. Training issues in emergency psychiatry. Psychiatr Clin North Am 1999;22(4):941–54.
8. Fauman BJ. Psychiatric residency training in the management of emergencies. Psychiatr Clin North Am 1983;6(2):325–34.
9. Lofchy J, Boyles P, Delwo J. Emergency psychiatry: clinical and training approaches. Can J Psychiatry 2015;60(6):1–7.
10. Bordage G, Harris I. Making a difference in curriculum reform and decision-making processes. Med Educ 2011;45(1):87–94.
11. Gallagher KA, Bujoreanu IS, Cheung P, et al. Psychiatric boarding in the pediatric inpatient medical setting: a retrospective analysis. Hosp Pediatr 2017;7(8):444–50.
12. Wharff EA, Ginnis KB, Ross AM, et al. Predictors of psychiatric boarding in the pediatric emergency department: implications for emergency care. Pediatr Emerg Care 2011;27(6):483–9.
13. Chien J, Sugar J, Shoemaker E, et al. Reflective team supervision after a frightening event on a psychiatric crisis service. Acad Psychiatry 2012;36(6):452–6.
14. Thomson AB, Cross S, Key S, et al. How we developed an emergency psychiatry training course for new residents using principles of high-fidelity simulation. Med Teach 2013;35(10):797–800.